MW00710255

LABORATORY PROFILES OF EQUINE DISEASES

LABORATORY PROFILES OF EQUINE DISEASES

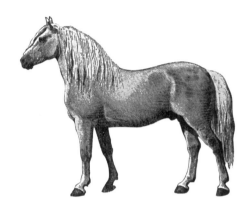

Susan C. Eades, D.V.M., Ph.D., Dip. A.C.V.I.M.

Department of Large Animal Medicine
College of Veterinary Medicine
University of Georgia
Athens, Georgia

Denise I. Bounous, D.V.M., Ph.D., Dip. A.C.V.P.

Department of Pathology
College of Veterinary Medicine
University of Georgia
Athens, Georgia

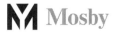 Mosby

St. Louis Baltimore Boston Carlsbad Chicago Naples New York Philadelphia Portland
London Madrid Mexico City Singapore Sydney Tokyo Toronto Wiesbaden

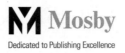

Mosby

Dedicated to Publishing Excellence

A Times Mirror
Company

Executive Editor: Paul W. Pratt, V.M.D.
Senior Developmental Editor: Jolynn Gower
Project Manager: Mark Spann
Production Editor: Stephen C. Hetager
Book Design Manager: Judi Lang
Graphic Design: Susan Vaughan Bongiorno,
    Jonathan Peck Typographers, Ltd.
Manufacturing Supervisor: Tony McAllister

Copyright © 1997 by Mosby–Year Book, Inc.

All rights reserved. No part of this publication may be reproduced, stored in a
retrieval system, or transmitted, in any form or by any means, electronic, mechani-
cal, photocopying, recording, or otherwise, without prior written permission from
the publisher.

Permission to photocopy or reproduce solely for internal or personal use is permit-
ted for libraries or other users registered with the Copyright Clearance Center, provided that the base fee of $4.00 per chapter plus $.10 per page is paid directly to the
Copyright Clearance Center, 27 Congress Street, Salem, MA 01970. This consent
does not extend to other kinds of copying, such as copying for general distribution,
for advertising or promotional purposes, for creating new collected works, or for
resale.

Printed in the United States of America.
Composition by Jonathan Peck Typographers, Ltd.
Printing/binding by R.R. Donnelley

Mosby–Year Book, Inc.
11830 Westline Industrial Drive
St. Louis, MO 63146

ISBN 0–8151–1731–0

96 97 98 99 00 / 9 8 7 6 5 4 3 2 1

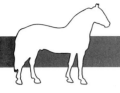

PREFACE

This book was written to provide easily accessible information about laboratory tests for equine patients. Laboratory medicine is an integral part of equine practice. Laboratory sources are widely available. Equine clinical texts provide information about laboratory tests within lengthy discussions of diseases. The format of this book facilitates rapid review.

Section 1 explains the use of various laboratory tests and differential diagnoses for changes in test results. Sections 2 and 3 present algorithms that begin with an abnormal laboratory result (Section 2) or clinical sign (Section 3) and provide a differential diagnosis and the appropriate laboratory tests used. Sections 4 to 14 present the clinical signs and laboratory profiles associated with nearly 80 equine diseases. Laboratory tests (Section 1), laboratory abnormalities (Section 2), and clinical signs (Section 3) are listed alphabetically. Diseases (Sections 4 to 14) are listed anatomically.

The reader may use this text by looking at a discussion of a specific disease to find the key tests performed to confirm a diagnosis. Alternatively, the index and algorithms may be consulted to find a differential diagnosis for abnormal laboratory test results. The discussions of the diseases that cause these laboratory abnormalities are then consulted to find a match with the observed profile. However, this book is not intended for use as the sole basis for diagnosis. History, clinical signs, and results of other diagnostic tests must be considered. Furthermore, laboratory changes listed in this text may not be observed in every case. Therefore, the laboratory profile should only be used as an aid to diagnosis.

The reference ranges provided were established in the clinical laboratory at the University of Georgia College of Veterinary Medicine or were compiled from multiple texts. Errors in interpretation can result from inappropriate reference ranges. *Readers are cautioned to use reference ranges established for their own laboratories.*

Susan C. Eades
Denise I. Bounous

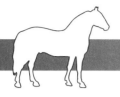

CONTENTS

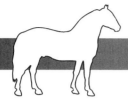

Significance of Laboratory Tests

Proteins

Albumin

Fibrinogen

Globulins

Total serum protein

Enzymes

Alanine aminotransferase (ALT)

Alkaline phosphatase (ALP)

Aspartate aminotransferase (AST)

Creatine kinase (CK)

Gamma-glutamyltransferase (GGT)

Lactate dehydrogenase (LDH)

Sorbitol dehydrogenase (SDH)

Other chemistry assays

Anion gap

Bile acids (BA)

Bilirubin

Calcium (Ca)

Chloride (Cl)

Creatinine

Glucose

Magnesium (Mg)

Phosphorus (P)

Potassium (K)

Sodium (Na)

Total CO_2 (tCO_2)

Urea nitrogen (SUN)

Hematology

Total WBC count

Basophils

Eosinophils

Lymphocytes

Monocytes

Neutrophils

Erythrocytes

Erythrocyte indices (MCV, MCH, MCHC)

Reticulocytes and nucleated RBC

Thrombocytes

Urinalysis

Urinary casts

Urine epithelial cells

Urine erythrocytes (RBC)

Urine leukocytes (WBC)

Urine glucose

Urine occult blood

Urine pH

Urine protein

Urine specific gravity

Endocrine tests

Cortisol

Dexamethasone suppression test

   Dexamethasone suppression screening test

   Standard dexamethasone suppression test

ACTH stimulation test

Combined dexamethasone suppression and
   ACTH stimulation test

Thyrotropin-releasing hormone (TRH) test

Thyroxine (T_4) and triiodothyronine (T_3)

Thyroid-stimulating hormone (TSH) test

Plasma testosterone concentration

Coagulation testing

ACT

APTT

FDP

OSPT

Fecal tests

Fecal blood

Fecal parasite examination

Response to anthemintic treatment

Salmonella culture of feces

Tests for rotavirus

Tests for sand

Serologic tests

Babesiosis

Borrelia burgdorferi infection (Lyme disease)

Eastern and western encephalitis

Ehrlichiosis

Equine herpesvirus infection

Equine infectious anemia (EIA)

Equine protozoal myelitis (*Sarcocystis falcatula* infection)

Equine viral arteritis (EVA)

Influenza

Potomac horse fever

Special tests

Bone marrow aspiration

Coombs' test

D-glucose and D-xylose absorption tests

Fractional urinary excretion of electrolytes

Fractional urinary excretion of enzymes

Hyperkalemic periodic paralysis (HPP)

Serum iron and iron-binding capacity

Submaximal exercise challenge test

Sulfobromophthalein (BSP) clearance test

Water deprivation test
CSF albumin and immunoglobulin

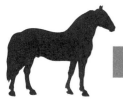

SIGNIFICANCE OF LABORATORY TESTS

This section describes the most common and useful hematology, chemistry, and special tests, followed by a list of the most common differential diagnoses for abnormal results. The tests included are by no means an exhaustive list. The discussions are designed to assist with interpretation of abnormal test results. However, test results always must be interpreted with clinical signs and physical findings for an accurate diagnosis.

Careful consideration should be given to collection and submission of blood samples for all laboratory tests. Artifactual or misleading laboratory data can be the result of mishandling. The laboratory can be consulted before sample submission for instructions on collection and handling. Samples for hematology tests are generally collected in EDTA. Anticoagulated whole blood should never be allowed to freeze, because red blood cell lysis will occur. Chemistry tests are generally performed on serum. It is necessary to remove the serum from clotted blood specimens as soon as possible, particularly if there is any delay in delivery to the laboratory.

The reference ranges provided were established in the clinical laboratory at the University of Georgia College of Veterinary Medicine or were compiled from multiple texts. Errors in interpretation can result from inappropriate reference ranges. Differences in assay technique can produce wide variation in test results. *Readers are cautioned to use reference ranges established for their own laboratories.*

PROTEINS

Albumin

↓ with intestinal malabsorption, malnutrition/starvation, chronic inflammatory disease, chronic liver disease, glomerulonephritis, nephrotic syndrome

↑ only with severe dehydration

Albumin Albumin is the most important component for maintaining plasma oncotic pressure. It binds and transports other proteins, amino acids, hormones, and drugs. Albumin is selectively lost in renal disease (glomerulonephritis, tubular damage, nephrotic syndrome) and gastrointestinal disease. Hypoalbuminemia resulting from decreased synthesis is associated with intestinal malabsorption, malnutrition/starvation, chronic inflammatory disease, and chronic liver disease. Increased albumin concentration occurs only in severe dehydration.

Reference range: 2.6 to 4.1 g/dl
Our laboratory's range:
_____

Fibrinogen [2, 45]
↑ with inflammation
↓ with DIC, liver failure, major surgery

Fibrinogen Fibrinogen functions in blood coagulation and to contain inflammatory conditions. Plasma concentration is increased in inflammation and decreased in disseminated intravascular coagulation, hepatic failure, and major surgery.

> Reference range: 100 to 400 mg/dl
> Our laboratory's range:

Globulins [2, 45]
↑ with chronic inflammatory disease, immune-mediated disease

monoclonal gammopathies seen with multiple myeloma, sometimes lymphomas

↓ with failure of passive transfer, CID, IgM deficiency, severe total protein loss

Globulins Globulins are composed of alpha-, beta-, and gamma-globulin fractions. Lipoproteins and acute-phase proteins migrate as alpha-globulins; complement and iron-containing proteins migrate in the beta-globulin region; immunoglobulins are the important component of the gamma-globulins. Alpha-globulins are often increased after tissue injury or acute inflammation. Increases in beta-globulins alone are unusual, but beta-globulins can often be increased in association with hypergammaglobulinemia of an intense immune response. Gamma-globulins are increased as a polyclonal gammopathy in cases of chronic inflammatory diseases, immune-mediated diseases, and some lymphoid neoplasms, and as monoclonal gammopathies with multiple myeloma or lymphoid neoplasm.

> Reference range: 2.6 to 4.0 g/dl
> Our laboratory's range:

Total serum protein [2, 39, 45]
↑ with dehydration, inflammation, multiple myeloma
↓ with renal disease, GI disease, liver failure, starvation

Total serum protein Total serum protein is composed of albumin and globulins and may vary depending on changes in any of these components. Total protein must be evaluated in relation to albumin concentration; for example, although total protein may decrease in the face of hypoalbuminemia, a concurrent hyperglobulinemia may cause the total protein to remain within the reference range. In general, increases in total protein may be seen with dehydration, septic or nonseptic inflammation, and myeloma. Decreases resulting from loss are seen with renal and gastrointestinal diseases; hepatic disease and starvation may result in decreased production.

> Reference range: 5.6 to 7.6 g/dl
> Our laboratory's range:

ENZYMES

Alanine aminotransferase (ALT) Hepatic ALT is very low in horses, and therefore not useful in detecting liver disease.

ALP [2, 45]
↑ with cholestasis, pregnancy, bone growth

Alkaline phosphatase (ALP) ALP isoenzymes are in every tissue, but ALP activity in healthy horses is primarily of hepatic origin. It is bound to intracellular microsomal enzymes. Cholestasis causes induction of hepatic ALP with increased serum activity. Serum ALP activity is usually normal or only mildly increased in acute hepatitis with very high serum

Readers are cautioned to use reference ranges established for their own laboratories.

AST activity. Placental ALP activity may be found in serum from healthy pregnant mares, and young growing animals have high activity.

Aspartate aminotransferase (AST) This enzyme occurs in almost all cells, but is used as a diagnostic enzyme for liver and muscle disease because of its high activity in these tissues. AST increases with changes, such as sublethal injury and necrosis, in muscle and hepatocellular permeability. The plasma half-life of AST (approximately 18 hours) is longer than the half-life of creatine kinase (CK). Increased serum activity may persist for 7 to 10 days following liver or muscle damage. Increases in AST and CK activity indicate muscle damage; increases in AST and SDH activity indicate liver damage.

AST [2, 45]
↑ with liver disease, when accompanied by ↑ SDH, or muscle disease, when accompanied by ↑ CK activity

> Reference range: 160 to 412 U/L
> Our laboratory's range:
> _____

Creatine kinase (CK) CK isoenzymes are found in skeletal (CKMM) and cardiac muscle (CKMB) and brain (CKBB). Isoenzyme testing is an important diagnostic tool for differentiation of cardiac disease. Total serum CK enzyme activity is derived from skeletal and cardiac muscle. Increases in total serum CK activity are associated with primary muscle diseases characterized by degeneration or necrosis, or secondary to vascular impairment, such as in vasculitis, or extreme shock. Muscular atrophy, neoplasia, or ischemic injury without associated degeneration or necrosis will not cause increases. A significant artifactual increase in serum CK activity may occur with hemolysis, excess bilirubin, or muscle fluid associated with difficult venipuncture. Moderate increases may accompany transport, periodic hyperkalemia, and strenuous exercise. However, increases of more than 500 IU within 2 hours after exercise indicate poor adaptation to training. Extremely high serum CK activity may be seen with exertional rhabdomyolysis or nutritional muscular dystrophy. The plasma half-life of CK in horses is short (about 2 hours).

CK [2, 45]
↑ with muscle necrosis

> Reference range: 60 to 330 U/L
> Our laboratory's range:
> _____

Gamma-glutamyltransferase (GGT) GGT is associated primarily with microsomal enzymes and, to a lesser degree, with the cellular cytosol. The canalicular surfaces of hepatocytes and bile duct epithelium and renal convoluted tubular cells contain the greatest activity. Serum GGT activity increases with cholestasis, and secondarily with hepatocellular damage. A mild to moderate increase in serum GGT activity occurs with obstructive diseases of the large colon. Increased urine GGT-creatinine ratios are seen in acute renal failure.

GGT [2, 45]
↑ with cholestasis

> Reference range: 6 to 32 U/L
> Our laboratory's range:
> _____

Readers are cautioned to use reference ranges established for their own laboratories.

Lactate dehydrogenase (LDH) Serum LDH activity is nonspecific; however, muscle, liver, and erythrocytes are sources of high activity. In horses, increases in serum LDH activity are not specific and are not useful in diagnosis.

SDH [2, 45]

↑ with hepatic injury or necrosis

Sorbitol dehydrogenase (SDH) SDH activity is high in the hepatocellular cytosol, and increased serum SDH activity indicates acute change in hepatocellular permeability associated with hepatic injury or necrosis. Increases have also been seen with obstructive or strangulating gastrointestinal lesions and acute enterocolitis caused by bacterial toxins from the damaged bowel entering portal circulation. Mild increases may be seen with anoxia from shock, acute anemia, or anesthesia. The half-life is short (a few hours), and continued increased activity indicates ongoing liver damage.

Reference range: 1 to 8 U/L
Our laboratory's range:

OTHER CHEMISTRY ASSAYS

AG [2, 42, 45]

↑ with metabolic acidosis

↓ occurs with hemodilution, hypoalbuminemia

Anion gap The anion gap is a calculated value of all unmeasured serum cations minus all unmeasured serum anions: $AG = [(Na^+ + K^+) - (Cl^- + HCO_3^-)]$. Most changes occur because of changes in unmeasured anions, such as small organic anions, albumin, and exogenous toxins. Increased anion gap occurs in many diseases, including lactic acidosis and renal insufficiency. Decreased anion gap rarely occurs; it may be seen with hemodilution and hypoalbuminemia.

Reference range: 0 to 9
Our laboratory's range:

Bile acids [2, 45]

↑ indicates decreased liver function

Bile acids (BA) Bile acid formation is the major endstage of cholesterol metabolism. Bile acids circulate through the intestines, into the portal circulation, and return to the liver, where the cycle begins again. Measurement of total serum bile acids is commonly used to evaluate liver disease in conjunction with bilirubin concentration and serum enzyme activities. Fasting levels less than 20 μmol/L are usual, with concentrations greater than 20 μmol/L occurring in hepatopathies associated with decreased liver function.

Reference range: 0 to 20 μmol/L
Our laboratory's range:

Bilirubin Bilirubin is derived from hemoglobin catabolism of senescent erythrocytes and from nonheme porphyrins. Equine hyperbilirubinemia is predominantly indirect (unconjugated). Hyperbilirubinemia associated with hemolysis typically is less than 25% direct (conjugated). Hyperbilirubinemia associated with intrahepatic or extrahepatic obstruction usually is 15% to 40% direct (conjugated). Hyperbilirubinemia of

Readers are cautioned to use reference ranges established for their own laboratories.

neonatal isoerythrolysis in foals may reach 20 mg/dl and may be largely direct. Anorexia is a common cause of hyperbilirubinemia in horses. The total bilirubin in these cases may reach 12 mg/dl, with the direct fraction remaining within the normal absolute range.

Reference range: Total 0.0 to 3.2 mg/dl
Direct 0.0 to 0.4 mg/dl
Our laboratory's range:

Calcium (Ca) Calcium is present in the plasma in three forms: protein-bound calcium, complexed calcium, and ionized calcium. About 50% of calcium is bound to protein. Serum calcium is reported as total calcium. Diet, albumin, and endogenous hormone concentrations influence calcium concentration. Parathormone (PTH) promotes renal tubular reabsorption of calcium and increases net rate of bone resorption and intestinal absorption of dietary calcium. Calcitonin is produced in response to hypercalcemia and regulates PTH resorptive action on bone. Vitamin D promotes calcium resorption by the intestinal mucosa. Hypercalcemia may occur in cases of hyperparathyroidism, neoplasms (gastric squamous cell carcinoma, malignant lymphoma), hypervitaminosis D (plant intoxication), excess calcium intake, chronic renal disease, and maximal exercise. Hypocalcemia can occur with hypoalbuminemia, cantharidin (blister beetle) toxicosis, lactation tetany, transport tetany, acute renal failure, decreased intake, gastrointestinal disease, and excess sweating.

Reference range: 10.2 to 13.4 mg/dl
Our laboratory's range:

Calcium [2, 38, 39, 43, 44, 45]

↑ with hyperparathyroidism, some neoplasms, hypervitaminosis D, excessive calcium intake, chronic renal disease, maximal exercise

↓ with hypoalbuminemia, cantharidin toxicosis, lactation tetany, acute renal failure, decreased intake, GI disease, excessive sweating

Chloride (Cl) Chloride is the major extracellular fluid anion. Increases and decreases in chloride concentration may parallel changes in sodium concentration and vary inversely with bicarbonate concentration. Loss of gastric HCl (anterior enteritis, strangulating or nonstrangulating obstruction of the small intestine) and colonic Cl^- (colitis) leads to hypochloridemia.

Reference range: 98 to 109 mEq/L
Our laboratory's range:

Chloride [2, 45]

↓ indicates gastrointestinal loss of Cl^-

Creatinine Creatinine is a nonprotein nitrogenous substance that originates endogenously from muscle metabolism. Creatinine is excreted by glomerular filtration, and increased concentrations occur with decreased renal blood flow. Creatinine concentration is increased with prerenal, renal, or postrenal azotemia, and is more sensitive to these conditions than is serum urea nitrogen. Concentrations are influenced by muscle mass. Well-muscled animals, such as stallions and draft breeds, have creatinine concentrations in the upper reference range. Creatinine concentration is not significantly affected by diet and catabolic factors.

Reference range: 0.4 to 2.2 mg/dl
Our laboratory's range:

Creatinine [2, 39, 45]

↑ with prerenal, renal, and postrenal disease

Readers are cautioned to use reference ranges established for their own laboratories.

Glucose [2, 40, 45]

↑ with hyperadrenocorticism, hyperpituitarism

↓ with adrenocortical insufficiency, liver failure, exertional extreme, septicemia, starvation, malabsorption

Glucose Blood glucose concentration is influenced by diet, the hormones insulin and glucagon, and the removal of glucose in the circulation. Persistent hyperglycemia occurs in hyperadrenocorticism and hyperpituitarism (pituitary adenoma). A transient hyperglycemia may be seen postprandially, with catecholamine and glucocorticoid release associated with pain or fear, CNS disease, and transport or stress. Hypoglycemia may occur with adrenocortical insufficiency, liver failure, exertional extreme, septicemia, starvation, or malabsorption. Artifactual decreases in serum glucose concentration may result from *in vitro* glycolysis by erythrocytes.

> Reference range: 62 to 134 mg/dl
> Our laboratory's range:

Magnesium [2, 39, 45]

↑ with renal failure, maximal exercise

↓ with hypoaldosteronism, excessive sweating, intestinal disease

Magnesium (Mg) Serum magnesium concentrations are diet dependent. Magnesium functions as a cofactor for many enzymes in the body. Magnesium balance is primarily affected by intestinal absorption, renal excretion, and lactation. Hypomagnesemia may be seen with hypoaldosteronism, intestinal diseases, excess sweating, or cantharidin toxicosis. Hypermagnesemia may be seen in renal failure and maximal exercise.

> Reference range: 1.4 to 2.3 mg/dl
> Our laboratory's range:

Phosphorus [2, 39, 44, 45]

↑ with nutritional secondary hyperparathyroidism, acute renal failure

↓ with chronic renal failure, starvation, hyperparathyroidism

Phosphorus (P) Phosphorus is found associated with calcium in the skeleton and teeth. Phosphorus concentration is also influenced by diet and endogenous hormone concentrations. Suckling foals have a higher range. Increased serum phosphorus concentration occurs with nutritional secondary hyperparathyroidism and with acute renal failure. Serum phosphorus is decreased in chronic renal failure, starvation, and hyperparathyroidism.

> Reference range: 1.5 to 4.7 mg/dl
> Our laboratory's range:

Potassium [2, 42, 45]

↑ with acidemia, maximal exercise, tissue necrosis, insulin deficiency, oliguria, uroperitoneum, adrenal insufficiency, hereditary periodic hyperkalemia

↓ with alkalemia, anorexia, excessive losses

Potassium (K) The concentration of intracellular fluid (ICF) potassium is higher than the concentration in extracellular fluid (ECF). Serum potassium is not a reliable indicator of total body potassium because shifts occur between ICF and ECF. Interpretation of total body potassium concentration must be made with reference to blood pH and the disease process. Hyperkalemia occurs with acidemia, maximal exercise, tissue necrosis, insulin deficiency, oliguria, uroperitoneum, adrenal insufficiency, and hereditary periodic hyperkalemia of Quarter horses. False hyperkalemia may result from erythrocyte hemolysis. Hypokalemia

Readers are cautioned to use reference ranges established for their own laboratories.

may result from depletion of body stores or from redistribution into the ICF. Hypokalemia can occur with alkalemia, anorexia, gastrointestinal losses, excess sweating, and urinary loss.

> Reference range: 2.9 to 4.6 mEq/L
> Our laboratory's range:

Sodium (Na) The majority of the body's sodium is found in the extracellular fluid. The remaining concentration of this cation is bound in skeletal bone. Sodium balance is controlled by changes in water balance and aldosterone. Aldosterone enhances sodium resorption in the kidney. Hypernatremia can occur with dehydration and salt poisoning. Hyponatremia is associated with diarrhea, excessive sweat losses, adrenal insufficiency, sequestration of fluid, and renal disease. Hyponatremia with hyperkalemia may accompany uroperitoneum and adrenal insufficiency.

> Reference range: 128 to 142 mEq/L
> Our laboratory's range:

Sodium [2, 45]

↑ with dehydration, salt poisoning

↓ with diarrhea, excessive sweat losses, adrenal insufficiency, fluid sequestration, renal disease

---

Total CO_2 (tCO_2) HCO_3 is the major component of tCO_2, and changes in tCO_2 are interpreted as changes in HCO_3. Decreased tCO_2 concentration indicates metabolic acidosis, and an increase in concentration indicates alkalosis.

> Reference range: 22 to 33 mEq/L
> Our laboratory's range:

tCO_2 [2, 45]

↑ indicates metabolic alkalosis

↓ indicates metabolic acidosis

Urea nitrogen (SUN) Urea nitrogen is synthesized in the liver from ammonia and excreted by glomerular filtration. Azotemia is an excess of urea or other nitrogenous products in the blood. Moderate increases in concentration of SUN are significant in the horse. Increased concentration of SUN is associated with decreased renal clearance as occurs with primary renal disease, prerenal or postrenal disease, and protein catabolism. Prerenal azotemia results from a decreased renal blood flow without functional change of the kidney. A concentrated urine (specific gravity ≥1.020), with urine osmolality three times greater than serum osmolality, absence of enzymuria, and low urine sodium concentrations, is expected with prerenal azotemia. Urea nitrogen concentration can also be affected by diet or by movement into extracellular fluid areas like the gastrointestinal tract. Postrenal azotemia occurs with obstruction to urine outflow or with a ruptured bladder. Decreased SUN concentration may occur with low-protein diet, liver failure, and anabolic steroids.

> Reference range: 11 to 27 mg/dl
> Our laboratory's range:

SUN [2, 45]

↑ with prerenal, renal, and postrenal disease, protein catabolism

↓ with liver failure, low-protein diet, anabolic steroid use

Readers are cautioned to use reference ranges established for their own laboratories.

HEMATOLOGY

Total WBC count The total number of WBC is increased or decreased by the numbers of neutrophils, lymphocytes, eosinophils, monocytes, and basophils.

> **Reference range:** 5.6 to 12.1 $\times$ 10^3/μl
> **Our laboratory's range:**

Basophils[2, 3]

basophil numbers rarely abnormal

Basophils Basophils are rarely seen in the peripheral blood of horses. Basophilia has been seen with allergic dermatitis.

> **Reference range:** 0 to 0.3 $\times$ 10^3/μl
> **Our laboratory's range:**

Eosinophils [2, 3]

rarely $\uparrow$ with parasitism

Eosinophils Eosinophilia may rarely accompany parasitic infections and allergic respiratory disease. However, intestinal parasitism and visceral larval migration (large strongyles and ascarids) rarely elicit a peripheral eosinophilia in horses. Eosinophilic granulocytic leukemia has been rarely reported in horses. Eosinopenia is difficult to evaluate, since eosinophil numbers are usually low in leukograms of normal horses.

> **Reference range:** 0 to 0.78 $\times$ 10^3/μl
> **Our laboratory's range:**

Lymphocytes [2, 3]

$\uparrow$ with excitement, exercise

$\downarrow$ with stress, glucocorticords, severe infection, endotoxemia, immunodeficiency, viral disease

Lymphocytes Physiologic lymphocytosis associated with excitement or exercise occurs commonly in horses under 2 years of age. Causes of lymphopenia include stress, exogenous corticosteroid administration, endotoxemia, severe bacterial infection, viral disease, and immunodeficiency.

> **Reference range:** 1.16 to 5.1 $\times$ 10^3/μl
> **Our laboratory's range:**

Monocytes [2, 3]

$\uparrow$ with chronic inflammation

Monocytes Monocytosis uncommonly occurs with chronic suppurative and granulomatous inflammation.

> **Reference range:** 0 to 0.7 $\times$ 10^3/μl
> **Our laboratory's range:**

Neutrophils [2, 3]

$\uparrow$ with stress, excitement, glucocorticoids, bacterial infection, neoplasia

$\downarrow$ with bacterial sepsis and endotoxemia

Neutrophils Stress, excitation, and exercise cause endogenous catecholamine release, resulting in a transient neutrophilia because of mobilization of the marginal neutrophil pool. Exogenous corticosteroid administration and endogenous corticosteroid release also cause neutrophilia. Acute bacterial infection, neoplasia, and other causes of tissue destruction (e.g., surgery) are pathologic causes of neutrophilia. Chronic localized bacterial infections are rarely accompanied by mild increases in neutrophil numbers. Recovery from endotoxemia may result in a

Readers are cautioned to use reference ranges established for their own laboratories.

rebound neutrophilia. The most common causes of neutropenia are bacterial sepsis and endotoxemia as large numbers of neutrophils leave the circulating pool and marginate to the vascular endothelium. During severe inflammatory diseases, large numbers of neutrophils leave the circulation to the site of tissue injury. Bone marrow dysfunction and neoplasia are rare causes of neutropenia. Bacterial infection, bacteremia, and endotoxemia may also increase the number of immature or band neutrophils in the circulation. Neutrophil morphology can be extremely helpful in determining the presence of bacterial infections that can result in neutrophil cytoplasmic changes referred to as "toxic changes." These include cytoplasmic vacuolation, basophilia, Dohle bodies, and "toxic" granulation.

> **Reference range:** segmented 2. 9 to 8.5 $\times$ 10^3/μl
> band 0 to 0.1 $\times$ 10^3/μl
> **Our laboratory's range:**

Erythrocytes A deficiency of RBC can be caused by blood loss, hemolysis, parasitism, renal failure, chronic inflammatory diseases, and rarely hematopoietic malignances. Polycythemia is usually relative, resulting from dehydration or splenic contraction. Absolute polycythemia usually is secondary to tissue hypoxia at high altitudes, chronic pulmonary disease, or heart defects. Inappropriate secondary erythrocytosis resulting from hepatocellular carcinoma has been rarely reported in horses.

Equine erythrocytes are retained in the bone marrow until hemoglobin synthesis is complete. Thus, polychromasia and macrocytosis are extremely rare in horses. Howell-Jolly bodies can occur in a small number of erythrocytes in healthy horses and do not represent young cells in the peripheral blood. Rouleaux formation is common for equine erythrocytes. This sometimes must be differentiated from autoagglutination by dilution (1 to 4) with saline solution.

> **Reference range:** 6 to 10.43 $\times$ 10^6/μl
> **Our laboratory's range:**

Erythrocytes[2, 3]
↓ with blood loss, hemolysis, chronic inflammation, bone marrow neoplasia
↑ with dehydration or splenic contraction

Erythrocyte indices (MCV, MCH, MCHC) Macrocytosis (increased MCV) indicates release of immature RBC from the bone marrow during regeneration, which is very rare in horses. Microcytosis (decreased MCV) caused by iron deficiency occurs occasionally in horses. An increased MCH usually indicates hemolysis, and a decreased MCH usually indicates iron deficiency. An increased MCHC will result from hemolysis, and a decreased MCHC may result from iron deficiency.

> **Reference range:** MCV   37 to 49 fl
> MCH   13.7 to 18.2 pg
> MCHC 35.3 to 39.3 g/dl
> **Our laboratory's range:**

Erythrocyte indices[2, 3]
MCV rarely ↑ with regenerative anemia
MCHC, MCV, and MCH rarely ↓ with iron deficiency
↑ MCH and MCHC indicate hemolysis

Readers are cautioned to use reference ranges established for their own laboratories.

Reticulocytes and nucleated RBC [2, 3]

not seen in equine peripheral blood

Reticulocytes and nucleated RBC Reticulocytes are immature RBC with a fine reticulum of nucleotide material that stains with methylene blue. Nucleated RBC are large and more immature than reticulocytes and erythrocytes. In other species, these cells are released into the peripheral blood during regeneration of anemia. Equine erythrocytes are retained in the bone marrow until maturity; therefore, the appearance of these cells in the peripheral blood is rare.

> Reference range: 0
> Our laboratory's range:

Thrombocytes [2, 3]

↓ with DIC, immune-mediated thrombocytopenia, EIA, ehrlichiosis, lymphosarcoma, excessive clumping in EDTA

Thrombocytes Decreased numbers of circulating platelets may result from disseminated intravascular coagulation, immune-mediated thrombocytopenia, endotoxemia, equine infectious anemia, equine ehrlichiosis, or lymphosarcoma. Severe hemorrhage (due to DIC) may cause thrombocytopenia. Platelets sometimes clump excessively in EDTA, thereby artifactually decreasing the count.

> Reference range: 117 to 256 $\times$ 10^3/μl
> Our laboratory's range:

URINALYSIS

Urinary casts [2, 3]

indicate renal tubular disease

Urinary casts Casts are cylindric accumulations of protein and cellular debris that form in the renal tubules. Casts may consist of RBC, WBC, or renal tubular epithelial cells. Hyaline casts are formed from mucoprotein resulting from glomerulonephritis or severe nephropathy. When present in the urine, casts indicate renal tubular disease. However, the number of casts does not necessarily correlate with the severity of disease.

Urine epithelial cells [2, 3]

↑ with renal tubular or urinary tract disease

Urine epithelial cells Epithelial cells in urine may be squamous, transitional, or renal tubular. The presence of small numbers of epithelial cells in urine is normal; however, large numbers may accompany renal tubular or urinary tract inflammation or neoplasia.

Urine erythrocytes [2, 3]

↑ with neoplasia, calculi, inflammation, coagulopathy

Urine erythrocytes (RBC) An increased number of RBC (greater than 5 per high-power field) indicates hematuria resulting from neoplasia, cystic or renal calculi, inflammation, acute tubular disease, or coagulopathy.

Urine leukocytes [2, 3]

↑ with genitourinary tract inflammation

Urine leukocytes (WBC) An increased number of WBC (greater than 5 per high-power field) indicates an inflammatory process in the genitourinary tract.

Urine glucose [2, 3]

↑ with stress, pituitary adenoma, diabetes mellitus

Urine glucose Although glucose is not normally found in the urine, when the blood glucose exceeds the urine threshold (160 to 180 mg/dl), glucosuria occurs. Causes of hyperglycemia and glucosuria include

---

Readers are cautioned to use reference ranges established for their own laboratories.

pituitary adenoma, diabetes mellitus, and catecholamine and glucocorticoid hormone release resulting from stress.

Urine occult blood   A positive reaction on urine dipsticks does not differentiate between hematuria, myoglobinuria, and hemoglobinuria. Hematuria clears after sedimentation or centrifugation and is accompanied by an increased number of red blood cells per high-power field. Myoglobinuria tends to produce a brown color and can be confirmed by chemical methods. Hematology can help in differentiation of hemoglobinuria and myoglobinuria. Hemoglobinemia is accompanied by anemia and frequently discolors the plasma red. Myoglobinemia is not accompanied by discoloration of plasma.

Urine pH   The pH of urine in adult horses is usually alkaline (7 to 9). Foals usually have slightly acidic urine (pH < 7). Aciduria in adult horses may be seen after exertional exercise, after prolonged fasting, or in response to metabolic acidosis. Hypokalemia may result in paradoxical aciduria. Renal tubular acidosis, in which patients excrete alkaline urine despite systemic acidosis, has been rarely diagnosed.

Urine protein   Protein is not normally found in the urine. With alkaline urine, false-positive protein reactions occur on urine dipsticks. Therefore, urine with a positive reaction on dipsticks should be checked by an acid precipitation procedure. Hemorrhage (cystic calculi, neoplasia, trauma from catheterization, clotting abnormalities, etc.) or inflammation (pyelonephritis, cystitis, genital infection, vasculitis, etc.) in the urogenital tract may cause proteinuria. Persistent, strong reactions for protein without evidence of hemorrhage or inflammation are indicative of glomerular disease (glomerulonephritis or amyloidosis).

Urine specific gravity   Specific gravity is a measure of the kidney's ability to concentrate and dilute urine. Normal animals have the ability to dilute their urine specific gravity to less than 1.008 and to concentrate the specific gravity to greater than 1.020. Neonatal foals usually have a urine specific gravity of less than 1.010 because of their high volume of fluid intake. Renal failure results in tubular dysfunction and isosthenuria (specific gravity 1.008 to 1.012). Failure to produce a concentrated urine (<1.020) in the face of dehydration also rarely results from diabetes insipidus.

ENDOCRINE TESTS

Cortisol   Cortisol is produced by the adrenal cortex and is an important modulator of many cellular functions. Therefore, adrenocortical dysfunction can result in numerous metabolic alterations. Serum cortisol

---

Urine occult blood[2, 3]
↑ from erythrocytes, myositis, hemolysis

Urine pH[2, 3]
↓ may indicate metabolic acidosis or hypokalemia
↓ or ↑ with renal tubular acidosis

Urine protein[2, 3]
↑ from glomerulonephritis, urinary or renal hemorrhage, inflammation, false reaction caused by alkalinity

Urine specific gravity[2, 3]
isosthenuria from renal failure

Cortisol[7-10]
↑ with stress or pituitary adenoma
↓ with adrenal insufficiency

Readers are cautioned to use reference ranges established for their own laboratories.

concentrations reflect adrenocortical function and can be decreased in horses with adrenal insufficiency and increased in horses with pituitary adenoma (Cushing's disease). However, horses with these diseases can often have normal serum cortisol concentrations. Serum cortisol levels also may be elevated in response to stress. Therefore, when adrenal insufficiency or pituitary adenoma (Cushing's disease) is suspected, ACTH stimulation and dexamethasone suppression tests, respectively, should be performed.

Reference range:	**3 to 13 µg/dl**
Adrenal insufficiency	**< 1 µg/dl**
Stress or pituitary adenoma	**>13 µg/dl**

Dexamethasone suppression test [7-10]

partial or transient suppression with pituitary adenoma

Dexamethasone suppression test Cortisol secretion is regulated by pituitary ACTH production. Normally, rising circulating cortisol concentration and administration of dexamethasone inhibit pituitary ACTH release. In horses with normal pituitary function, dexamethasone administration will result in a sustained decrease in serum cortisol concentration. In horses with pituitary adenoma, dexamethasone administration may cause incomplete suppression of cortisol release. That is, suppression of cortisol production in horses with pituitary disease may be partial (>1 µg/dl) or transient (<1 µg/dl for less than 24 hours). The dexamethasone screening test or standard protocol may be used.

Dexamethasone suppression screening test [7-10]

partial or transient suppression with pituitary adenoma

Dexamethasone suppression screening test This protocol provides an excellent screening test for horses suspected to have pituitary adenoma. A blood sample is collected in a heparinized container at 4 to 6 P.M. Dexamethasone is administered at 40 µg/kg intramuscularly, and a heparinized blood sample is collected at noon the following day.

Reference range:	
Posttreatment cortisol concentration	**< 1 µg/dl**
Pituitary adenoma	**>1 µg/dl**

Standard dexamethasone suppression test [7-10]

partial or transient suppression with pituitary adenoma

Standard dexamethasone suppression test Because it incorporates more extensive sampling times than does the screening test, this standard protocol allows more precise assessment of pituitary function. A pretest blood sample is collected in a heparinized container at midnight. Dexamethasone is administered at 40 µg/kg intramuscularly. Heparinized blood samples are collected at 8 A.M., noon, 4 P.M., 8 P.M., and midnight.

Reference range:	
Posttreatment cortisol concentration	
by 18 to 24 hours after cortisol	**<1 µg/dl**
Pituitary adenoma (Cushing's disease)	
for all posttreatment times	
after 18 to 24 hours	**>1 µg/dl**

Readers are cautioned to use reference ranges established for their own laboratories.

ACTH stimulation test The ACTH stimulation test is used to identify horses with adrenal insufficiency. A heparinized blood sample is collected between 8 and 10 A.M. ACTH gel (1 IU/kg intramuscularly) or synthetic ACTH (100 IU intravenously) is administered. A post-ACTH blood sample is collected at 2 and 4 hours (ACTH gel) or at 2 hours (synthetic ACTH) after ACTH administration.

ACTH stimulation test [7-10]
↓ response indicates adrenal insufficiency

> Reference range:
> Posttreatment cortisol   2 to 3 times increase
> Adrenal insufficiency   less than 2 times increase

Combined dexamethasone suppression and ACTH stimulation test This test is not useful in horses, since it does not allow sufficient time to assess complete suppression of pituitary ACTH production after dexamethasone administration.

Combined dexamethasone suppression and ACTH stimulation test [7-10]
Usually nondiagnostic

Thyrotropin-releasing hormone (TRH) test TRH will stimulate ACTH secretion when there is pituitary disease. A pretest blood sample is collected in a heparinized container. TRH is administered at a dose of 1 mg intravenously. Heparinized blood samples are collected before and 0.25, 0.5, 1, 1.5, 2, and 3 hours after TRH administration. Plasma samples are assayed for cortisol.

Thyrotropin-releasing hormone (TRH) test [4-10]
↑ cortisol suggests pituitary adenoma

> Reference range:
> Pituitary adenoma   Cortisol > baseline

Thyroxine (T_4) and triiodothyronine (T_3) Circulating concentrations of thyroid hormones are sometimes used as a measure of thyroid function. Thyroxine (T_4) is the principal hormone produced by the thyroid gland; it is degraded in peripheral tissues to triiodothyronine (T_3), the more potent hormone. The majority of thyroid hormone is protein bound in circulation. The active forms (free T_3 and T_4) are not protein bound. Radioimmunoassays have been adapted to more accurately measure equine thyroid hormones. The serum concentration of T_4 in horses is one-fourth that in people. Therefore, special techniques are required to accurately assay thyroid hormone concentrations in horses.

Thyroxine (T_4) and triiodothyronine (T_3) [4-10]
↓ with hypothyroidism, pituitary adenoma, drug therapy, diet

   Insufficient production of thyroid hormone by the thyroid gland, deficiency of TSH produced by the pituitary gland, and decreased production of thyroid-releasing hormone by the hypothalamus can result in hypothyroidism. It has not been well documented that such functional hypothyroidism occurs in adult horses. Phenylbutazone administration, high-energy diets, high-protein diets, diets high in zinc and copper, glucocorticoid administration, fasting, and ingestion of endophyte-infected fescue grass can result in low concentrations of T_4 and T_3 in horses without disease. Therefore, plasma concentrations of T_4 and T_3 do not always

Readers are cautioned to use reference ranges established for their own laboratories.

provide a reliable method for diagnosis of hypothyroidism. In animals with abnormal serum concentrations of thyroid hormones, function should be evaluated with a TSH stimulation test.

	Reference range T_4 (mg/dl)	Reference range T_3 (ng/dl)
1.5 to 4 months	3 to 5.25	135 to 270
2 to 5 years	1.2 to 2.9	72 to 180
6 to 10 years	1.3 to 2.2	48 to 118
11 to 25 years	0.9 to 2.2	47 to 145

Thyroid-stimulating hormone

(TSH) test [4-10] ↓ with hypothyroidism

Thyroid-stimulating hormone (TSH) test Thyroid-stimulating hormone is produced by the pituitary gland and causes release of T_3 and T_4 from the thyroid gland. A pretest serum sample is collected and 5 IU of TSH is administered intramuscularly. A serum sample is collected at 1 hour and 4 hours after administration.

Reference range posttreatment	1 hr: 2 times increase in T_3
	4 hr: 2 times increase in T_3 and T_4
Hypothyroidism	<2 times increase

Plasma testosterone [9, 10]

↑ with pregnancy or granulosa-theca cell tumor

Plasma testosterone concentration The normal concentration of testosterone in plasma of nonpregnant mares is less than 50 pg/ml. During pregnancy, concentrations may exceed this value. Granulosa-theca cell tumors produce a variety of steroidal hormones, including testosterone. Plasma concentration of testosterone greater than 50 pg/ml in mares with compatible clinical findings is suggestive of a granulosa-theca cell tumor.

COAGULATION TESTING

Activated partial thromboplastin time (APTT) and one-stage prothrombin time (OSPT) are frequently evaluated in conjunction with platelet count and fibrinogen concentration.

Acquired deficiency of the vitamin K–dependent factors II, VII, IX, X occurs in coumarin/warfarin poisonings and results in prolongation of OSPT, APTT, and ACT. Animals with DIC usually exhibit prolonged APTT, OSPT, and ACT tests.

Horses with colic frequently have decreases in antithrombin III and protein C, which predispose them to hypercoagulation, but do not result in abnormal APTT, OSPT, or ACT.

ACT [2, 45]

prolonged with DIC, vitamin K deficiency, some factor deficiencies, thrombocytopenia

ACT Activated clotting time is a measure of intrinsic and common coagulation pathway function. The ACT is dependent on platelet

Readers are cautioned to use reference ranges established for their own laboratories.

phospholipid for activation, so that marked thrombocytopenia will result in prolongation of the ACT in the presence of normal concentrations of coagulation factors.

> Reference range: 120 to 190 seconds
> Our laboratory's range:

_____

APTT Activated partial thromboplastin time is the time required for fibrin clot formation after addition of a contact activator, phospholipid, and calcium to citrated plasma. Prolongation of APTT indicates deficiency in the intrinsic or common pathway of coagulation. Hereditary disorders of prekallikrein with prolongation of APTT alone have been reported in the horse.

> Reference range: 30 to 50 seconds
> Our laboratory's range:

_____

FDP Fibrin degradation products are the breakdown products of fibrinogen and fibrin that result from the activation of fibrinolysis. They can act as strong anticoagulants. Increases occur in patients with DIC or primary fibrinolysis. FDP are assayed using commercial reagents by detection of agglutination of latex particles coated with antibody to human fibrinogen fragments.

> Reference range: 0 to 16 mg/ml
> Our laboratory's range:

_____

OSPT The one-stage prothrombin time assay measures the time required for fibrin formation after the addition of tissue thromboplastin and calcium to citrated plasma. Prolongation of OSPT indicates deficiency in the extrinsic or common pathway of coagulation.

> Reference range: 8.2 to 11 seconds
> Our laboratory's range:

_____

FECAL TESTS

Fecal blood Numerous commercial tests, based upon the peroxidase activity of hemoglobin, are available for detection of hemoglobin in feces. Fecal blood can result from parasitism, gastric ulceration, enteritis or colitis, rectal trauma (manual examination), and drugs (nonsteroidal antiinflammatory drugs).

APTT [2, 45]
prolonged with DIC, some factor deficiencies, vitamin K deficiency, prekallikrein deficiency

FDP [2]
↑ with DIC, primary fibrinolysis

OSPT [2, 45]
prolonged with DIC, some factor deficiencies, vitamin K deficiency

Fecal blood [3, 9, 10]
↑ with parasitism, gastric ulceration, enterocolitis, NSAID use

Readers are cautioned to use reference ranges established for their own laboratories.

Fecal parasite examination [10-14]

↑ egg count with inadequate parasite control

Fecal parasite examination Qualitative (fecal flotation) and quantitative (McMaster or Wisconsin technique) analyses for parasite ova can be used to monitor the effectiveness of an endoparasite control program. Analysis of feces from 20% of the herd at 2 weeks after anthelmintic administration should not reveal parasite ova. Identification of parasite ova in more than 10% of samples is indication of resistance to the anthelmintic used. Examination of fecal samples from 20% of the horses should be repeated between dewormings. If egg counts increase to greater than 100 eggs per gram, the interval between dewormings should be decreased. The number of ova in fecal samples from 20% of the horses in the herd correlates with the amount of pasture contamination. However, quantitative fecal analysis does not correlate with the amount of disease caused by parasites in an individual horse. Furthermore, because the majority of intestinal damage is due to the larval stages, significant parasitism can exist with no parasite ova in feces. Therefore, fecal parasite examination is not useful for diagnosis of disease resulting from parasitism.

Protozoal agents sometimes are found in feces from horses. *Eimeria leukarti* is commonly shed by foals but does not cause disease. *Cryptosporidium* is an important cause of diarrhea in other species and occasionally is shed in feces of foals. However, it has not yet been associated with intestinal disease in foals. *Giardia equi* has been reported as a cause of diarrhea but the disease incidence is probably very low.

Response to anthelmintic treatment [10-14]

improved weight gain or fecal character after treatment indicates parasite-related disease

Response to anthelmintic treatment There are no specific laboratory tests to confirm the presence of intestinal disease resulting from parasitism. Parasitized horses do not develop peripheral eosinophilia resulting from parasitism. Abdominal fluid eosinophilia, hypergammaglobulinemia, abnormal palpation of the mesenteric vasculature, and high fecal ova counts are present in some horses with parasitism. However, these results do not correlate with severity of disease. Response to larvacidal anthelmintic treatment is used to confirm disease caused by parasitism. Larvacidal treatments used include fenbendazole (10 mg/kg daily for 5 days), fenbendazole (50 mg/kg daily for 3 days), ivermectin (200 µg/kg one dose), and oxfendazole. Improvement of clinical signs may take several weeks depending on the severity of the disease. It is sometimes necessary to repeat treatment every 30 days for 3 or 4 treatments.

Salmonella culture of feces [3, 9, 10]

positive with *Salmonella* infection

Salmonella culture of feces Successful culture of feces for *Salmonella* requires use of enrichment media to allow *Salmonella* to grow preferentially in place of the other enteric bacteria. In spite of these techniques, the organism is frequently not detected in the feces of animals shedding the organism intermittently or in low numbers. Increased sensitivity results from the culture of multiple fecal samples (minimum 5) or culture of tissues where the organism is harbored intracellularly (rectal mucosa, colonic mucosa and submucosa, mesenteric lymph node, liver).

Readers are cautioned to use reference ranges established for their own laboratories.

Tests for rotavirus Latex agglutination (virogen rotatest, Wampole Laboratories, Cranbury, New Jersey) and ELISA (Rotazyme II, Abbott Laboratories, North Chicago, Illinois) tests for rotaviral antigens are available commercially. These tests correlate well with virus detection by electron microscopy in several species, including horses.

Tests for sand Sand is heavier than ingesta and is detected by allowing it to settle out when water is added to feces. In some cases of impaction and colitis caused by sand, the sand settles in the intestine and is not passed. In these situations, administration of laxatives (water, psyllium, etc.) will initiate evacuation of sand in feces and allow it to be detected.

SEROLOGIC TESTS

Babesiosis Babesiosis is rarely diagnosed in most of the United States, but is endemic to Florida and Texas. Diagnosis is often made by demonstration of organisms in Giemsa- or Wright-stained blood smears. Since parasitemia precedes fever, parasitized RBCs may be removed before diagnostic testing is attempted. The complement fixation test for parasite antibodies is a more reliable diagnostic test. Horses usually seroconvert within 5 days of infection. Horses remain seropositive for 6 weeks to 8 months after eradication of the carrier state.

Borrelia burgdorferi **infection (Lyme disease)** Diagnosis of clinical Lyme disease is difficult and depends upon recognition of clinical signs, a history of possible exposure (ticks in endemic areas), confirmation of infection, absence of other disease, and response to treatment. Serologic testing is often the only practical means of confirming *B. burgdorferi* infection. Several assays for antibody detection have been developed. IFA is most widely used in domestic animals. There is not a standardized method of assay or an assessment of titers. It is important to select an experienced laboratory. Dogs and humans tend to develop higher titers than do horses and cattle. Spirochetes have been demonstrated by direct immunofluorescence in brain from a horse with ataxia, the anterior chamber of a pony with uveitis, and the kidneys and brain of fetuses from mares with stiffness, lameness, and reproductive failure. Serology from these horses revealed high IFA titers (1:1024 to 1:2048). Antibody has been found in synovial fluid of affected animals. CSF has not been tested for antibody in horses.

Eastern and western encephalitis Cerebrospinal fluid reveals increased WBC and RBC counts and total proteins in nearly all cases. However, lumbosacral CSF is sometimes normal when atlantooccipital CSF is abnormal. Neutrophils are the predominant cell type seen in the early phases of the disease, whereas lymphocytes predominate later. In many

Tests for rotavirus [3, 7, 15-17]

positive with rotavirus infection

Tests for sand [3, 7, 9, 10]

positive with intestinal sand accumulation

Test for babesiosis [10, 18, 19]

positive suggests horse is symptomatic or asymptomatic carrier

Borrelia burgdorferi **infection (Lyme disease)** [10, 20-23]

serology confirms exposure but not disease; immunofluorescence of tissues confirms disease

Eastern and western encephalitis [10, 24-26]

ratio of EEE:WEE titer >8, positive ELISA IgM titer, and virus isolation from brain confirm disease

Readers are cautioned to use reference ranges established for their own laboratories.

cases CSF eosinophil numbers are increased. Serology is sometimes a valuable indication of the presence of togavirus infection. Horses often do not survive long enough to allow for submission of paired serum samples. In the majority of horses with EEE infection the ratio of EEE titer to WEE titer is 8. In vaccinated horses without infection the ratio is low. Complement fixation and cross serum neutralization titers can be performed, and when their results are interpreted with results from CSF analysis and serologic titers, the chances of a positive diagnosis are increased. An ELISA can also differentiate vaccinal (IgG) and virus-induced (IgM) titers. CSF titers are frequently negative in affected horses. Virus isolation from brain tissue at postmortem is usually possible.

Ehrlichiosis [10, 27, 28]

serology confirms exposure, not disease; blood smear sometimes reveals organism

Ehrlichiosis Serology (indirect fluorescent antibody test) indicates exposure to the rickettsial organism, but does not confirm disease resulting from that exposure. Diagnosis is based on demonstration of characteristic organism in neutrophils and eosinophils with Giemsa or Wright stain of peripheral blood smears.

Equine herpesvirus infection [3, 10, 29]

virus isolation, paired serology, and CSF antibody can confirm disease

Equine herpesvirus infection Virus may be isolated from nasopharyngeal swabs and heparinized blood obtained as soon as possible after pyrexia is noticed. Nasal excretion of virus may be short lived, but cell-associated neuromas may last for weeks after infection. Detection of viral genome may be accomplished by use of the polymerase chain reaction in specialized laboratories.

Complement fixation and ELISA tests for measurement of antibody to EHV-1 and EHV-4 are available. Complement fixation titers rise and decline rapidly, so a high titer suggests recent exposure. Acute and convalescent sera from acutely infected animals often demonstrate a fourfold increase in titer. However, some animals fail to develop a strong antibody response. Some horses may not develop a peak titer until several weeks after infection.

Most horses with EHV-1 induced neurologic disease have high levels of antibody in the CSF. However, not all horses with signs of neurologic deficits and high CSF antibody titers have EHV-1 induced diseased. At postmortem, virus can often be isolated from the nervous system.

Serologic tests should not be used to diagnose EHV abortion. Examination of the fetus (especially lung, liver, thymus, adrenal gland) by histology (intranuclear inclusions), immunostaining, and virus isolation leads to diagnosis of EHV-1 abortion.

EIA [9, 10, 30]

positive test confirms infection

Equine infectious anemia (EIA) The serologic tests used for equine infectious anemia are agar gel immunodiffusion (Coggins) or competitive enzyme-linked immunoabsorbent assay (C-ELISA). Most horses will seroconvert by 40 days after infection and remain seropositive for life. The AGID and C-ELISA tests are recognized by the USDA as valid and

Readers are cautioned to use reference ranges established for their own laboratories.

reliable for the diagnosis of EIA. However, a few infected horses have had consistently negative AGID tests. AGID testing of CSF has provided the diagnosis in some neurologic cases.

Equine protozoal myelitis (*Sarcocystis falcatula* infection)   Western blot testing of serum and CSF antibody and polymerase chain reaction testing of protozoal DNA in CSF are being performed by Equine Biodiagnostics, Inc. (EBI), A153 ASTECC Building, University of Kentucky, Lexington, KY 40506-0286. Western blot testing of CSF appears to be specific and sensitive. False negatives rarely occur in very acute and very chronic cases. False positives may result from other insults to the blood-brain barrier allowing serum antibody to leak into the CSF. Positive serum titer confirms exposure, but not disease. However, very few horses with neurologic disease resulting from *Sarcocystis falcatula* are serum negative.

Equine protozoal myelitis [10, 31-33]

positive serum confirms exposure only; positive CSF suggests disease

Equine viral arteritis (EVA)   The serologic test most commonly used is serum neutralization. Acute infection is often confirmed by demonstrating a fourfold rising titer on serum samples obtained 3 to 4 weeks apart. Virus isolation may be attempted on nasopharyngeal swabs, heparinized blood, aborted fetus, or placenta. Identification of shedder stallions is made by virus isolation from semen or by seroconversion of negative mares after breeding.

Equine viral arteritis (EVA) [3, 9, 10]

virus isolation or paired serology confirms disease

Influenza   Influenza virus can be detected in nasal secretions by culture of infectious virus or by recognition of viral antigen (ELISA or IF). Nasopharyngeal swabs for virus culture should be collected within 48 hours of pyrexia and placed in virus transport media on ice to maintain virus viability. Immunostaining for virus antigen from nasopharyngeal swabs, tracheal washes, or nasal scrapings is sometimes more practical. Infection may be confirmed retrospectively by hemagglutination inhibition or single radial hemolysis testing of serum samples collected 14 to 21 days apart.

Influenza [3, 9, 10]

virus isolation or paired serology confirms disease

Potomac horse fever   Antibody to *Ehrlichia risticii* is measured by indirect fluorescent antibody testing. The test is useful for identification of endemic areas and for retrospective confirmation of the diagnosis. However, the test is not useful for directing therapy. A tendency toward false-positive or false-negative results limits the accuracy. Most horses develop antibody titers at the same time as or before occurrence of clinical signs. Paired serum samples should be collected 1 week apart. However, even with careful control of sample times, 50% of horses with the disease will have paired titers within 1 dilution of each other. These affected horses cannot be distinguished from those exposed (with titers over 1:5120). Potomac horse fever can be ruled out in horses with clinical signs of several days' duration with a negative titer.

Potomac horse fever [3, 9, 10]

paired serology sometimes confirms disease

Readers are cautioned to use reference ranges established for their own laboratories.

SPECIAL TESTS

Bone marrow aspiration [2]

↑ M:E ratio can indicate myeloid hyperplasia, erythroid hypoplasia

bone marrow iron can be ↓ with iron-deficiency anemia

bone marrow iron can be ↑ with anemia of chronic disease

Bone marrow aspiration Aspirates are usually obtained from the sternum, iliac crest, or ribs. Because equine reticulocytes are not found in the peripheral blood, a bone marrow aspiration may be indicated to determine whether anemia is regenerative. Finding ample numbers of polychromatic erythrocytes or reticulocytes in the bone marrow is a sign of effective erythropoiesis. Normal myeloid-to-erythroid ratios range from 0.5:1 to 1.5:1. Equine bone marrows normally contain stainable iron stores. Nonregenerative anemia of chronic disease is characterized by increased iron marrow stores. Marrow iron stores are decreased in iron-deficiency anemia.

Coombs' test Coombs' test is performed to aid in diagnosis of immune-mediated anemia. A direct Coombs test detects antibody and/or complement attached to the patient's cells. An indirect Coombs test detects antibody in the serum of the patient against erythrocytes. Agglutination following mixing of colostrum with the foal's blood detects maternal antibody to the foal's cells.

D-glucose and D-xylose absorption tests [3, 9, 10]

absent peak suggests malabsorption

D-glucose and D-xylose absorption tests These tests measure the small intestinal absorptive capacity. Mucosal cell damage, intestinal inflammation and edema, increased capillary hydrostatic pressure, and decreased plasma protein concentration are all abnormalities that might reduce small intestinal absorption. Acute diseases causing transient glucose and xylose malabsorption include strangulating and nonstrangulating obstruction, nonstrangulating infarction, and enteritis. Chronic diseases causing more persistent malabsorption include parasitism, enteric neoplasia, abdominal abscessation, and granulomatous, eosinophilic, basophilic, and lymphocytic enteritis. Cellular uptake and metabolism of glucose also affect the results of glucose absorption testing. Gastric emptying affects the results of both xylose and glucose absorption testing. Feed is withheld for 12 to 18 hours. Either D-glucose or D-xylose is administered at 0.5 g/kg in a 10% solution through a nasogastric tube. Blood is collected in sodium fluoride (glucose) or heparinized (xylose) tubes at 0, 30, 60, 90, 120, 150, 180, 210, and 240 minutes after administration.

Reference range	Peak 20 to 25 mg/dl at 60 to 120 min
Malabsorption	Depressed or absent peak
Delayed gastric emptying	Depressed or delayed peak

Fractional urinary excretion of electrolytes [3, 20, 34, 35]

renal disease ↑ FE of Na

potassium deficit ↓ FE of K

nutritional disease ↑ FE of P

Fractional urinary excretion of electrolytes Fractional urinary excretion of electrolytes can be calculated after simultaneous collection of urine and blood, and measurement of creatinine and electrolyte concentrations. The fractional excretion (FE) is calculated from the following formula:

$$FE = \frac{\text{Urine electrolyte}}{\text{Serum electrolyte}} \times \frac{\text{Serum creatinine}}{\text{Urine creatinine}} \times 100$$

Readers are cautioned to use reference ranges established for their own laboratories.

The fractional excretion of electrolytes is affected by tubular function, dietary intake, hormones, and drug therapy. In normal horses or horses with prerenal azotemia, the fractional excretion of sodium is less than 1%. Renal azotemia may increase the fractional excretion of sodium. Low fractional excretion of potassium may suggest a whole-body deficit of this electrolyte. Abnormal fractional excretion of phosphorus in an adult supports a diagnosis of hyperparathyroidism.

Healthy horses FE sodium	**<1%**
Renal azotemia	**>1%**
Healthy horses FE potassium	**15% to 65%**
Potassium deficit	**<15%**
Healthy horses FE phosphorus	**<1%**
Nutritional hyperparathyroidism	**>1%**

Fractional urinary excretion of enzymes   The urinary fractional excretion ratio of gamma-glutamyltransferase (GGT) can be calculated as indicated for electrolytes from simultaneously collected urine and serum samples after measurement of creatinine and GGT concentrations. Increased urinary enzyme activity has been associated with renal tubular disease and renal azotemia.

Healthy horses FE GGT	**<25%**
Renal disease	**>25%**

Fractional urinary excretion of enzymes [10, 36]

↑ with renal disease

Hyperkalemic periodic paralysis (HPP)   The DNA mutation for the membrane abnormality (HPP-type sodium channel) can be identified in susceptible horses. Testing is performed on EDTA-treated blood by the Veterinary Genetics Laboratory, School of Veterinary Medicine, Department of Medicine, University of California, Davis 95616-8737. Diagnosis in susceptible horses is based on clinical signs with an elevated serum potassium concentration. Other tests include electromyography (EMG) and oral potassium chloride challenge test. EMG changes indicate muscle disease, but are not specific. The potassium chloride challenge test involves oral administration of 0.1 g KCl/kg body weight. Positive diagnosis is based on clinical signs and hyperkalemia. This procedure is not recommended, because of the risk of death during an HPP attack and the availability of the blood test for identification of the HPP mutation.

Serum iron and iron-binding capacity   Free serum iron is minimal; however, lactoferrin and transferrin are serum carrier proteins that are normally 30% saturated with iron. The majority of iron is stored in tissues as hemoglobin, myoglobin, ferritin, and hemosiderin. Prussian blue staining of bone marrow is often performed to subjectively assess the amount of stored iron. A good-quality forage contains more than the necessary amount of dietary iron for horses. Therefore, iron-deficiency anemia is rare and only accompanies chronic severe blood loss. In this

Serum iron and iron-binding capacity [3]

↓ serum and marrow iron with ↑ binding capacity indicates iron deficiency

↓ serum iron and binding capacity with ↑ marrow iron indicates inflammation

Readers are cautioned to use reference ranges established for their own laboratories.

case serum iron is decreased, binding capacity is increased, and marrow iron stores are decreased. Inflammation is accompanied by a decrease in the serum iron. Furthermore, during the inflammatory response, neutrophils liberate lactoferrin, which transfers iron from transferrin to lactoferrin. Lactoferrin is taken up by macrophages to increase the storage of iron. Therefore, nonregenerative anemia of chronic disease is characterized by decreased serum iron, normal or decreased iron-binding capacity, and increased marrow iron stores.

Reference range:
Serum iron	70 to 140 mg/dl
Iron-binding capacity	200 to 262 mg/dl

Submaximal exercise challenge [10]

↑ CK at 24 hours after exercise indicates muscle disease

Submaximal exercise challenge test Measurement of CK activity in response to exercise can be used to assess muscular disorders. The half-life of CK is very short. Therefore, measurement of serum activity during periods of rest may not reflect mild damage or residual damage. An abnormal increase in CK activity after exercise indicates ongoing muscle damage probably resulting from underlying muscle disease. A blood sample is collected before exercise. Then, the horse is exercised submaximally (usually at trot or cantor) for 10 to 15 minutes. Blood samples are collected at 1, 6 and 24 hours after exercise. The CK activity should increase at 1 hour after exercise and return to normal by 6 to 24. Further increases in CK activity (from that obtained at 1 hour) at 6 and/or 24 hours indicate moderate to severe muscle disease. A decrease in CK activity at 24 hours with failure to return to normal indicates mild muscle disease.

Healthy horses	Increase at 1 hr, normal by 24 hr
Horses with muscle disease	Increase at 1 hr, still increased at 24 hr

Sulfobromophthalein (BSP) clearance [3, 9, 10]

↑ with liver failure

Sulfobromophthalein (BSP) clearance test The liver excretes a large number of exogenous compounds, and the rate of clearance of these substances can be used to test the liver's excretory function. The substance most commonly used in horses is BSP. The BSP clearance test is useful when results of bilirubin, bile acids, glucose, and SUN do not provide an adequate assessment of liver function. A heparinized blood sample is collected before injection. Sulfobromophthalein is injected intravenously at 2 mg/kg while care is taken to avoid perivascular injection. Heparinized blood samples are collected from the opposite jugular vein at 3, 5, 7, 9, and 12 minutes following injection. The laboratory assays the samples for BSP and determines the clearance half-life.

Reference range:	2.4 to 4.1 minutes
Liver failure	>4.1 minutes

Readers are cautioned to use reference ranges established for their own laboratories.

Water deprivation test   The water deprivation test allows differentiation of diabetes insipidus or renal failure from psychogenic polydipsia. Prolonged water deprivation is dangerous to azotemic animals or animals with persistent polyuria. In these cases water deprivation should be avoided or should be limited to a few hours with close monitoring. Failure to concentrate urine suggests central diabetes insipidus, renal disease, or medullary washout.

Protocol
1. Withhold water. Check urine specific gravity at 6 to 18 hours.
2. Provide water and terminate testing if urine specific gravity increases above 1.020, BUN or creatinine is increased, or the animal becomes dehydrated (tacky mucous membranes, increased PCV, TP).

Normal urine specific gravity	**>1.020**
Diabetes insipidus, medullary washout, renal failure	**<1.012**

Water deprivation test [2]

lack of urine concentration with renal disease

CSF albumin and immunoglobulin   The albumin quotient is the ratio of CSF albumin concentration to serum albumin concentration. An increased albumin quotient occurs with damage to the blood-brain barrier, as with equine herpesvirus encephalitis, trauma, or leakage during CSF sampling. Immunoglobulin G concentrations in the CSF are normally low but may increase from damage to the blood-brain barrier or as a result of intrathecal production in inflammatory neurologic disease. The IgG index is calculated from CSF IgG, serum IgG, CSF albumin, and serum albumin concentrations. The IgG index is increased in protozoal myelitis, polyneuritis equi, and cervical stenotic myelopathy. Samples may be submitted to Dr. Frank Andrew, Department of Rural Practice, P.O. Box 1071, Knoxville TN 37901-1071.

CSF albumin and immunoglobulin [37]

↑ albumin quotient with herpesvirus infection, trauma, or hemorrhage

↑ IgG index with protozoal myelitis

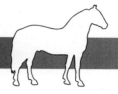
1. West HJ: Evaluation of total plasma bile acid concentrations for the diagnosis of hepatobiliary disease in horses, *Res Vet Sci* 46:254-270, 1989.

2. Duncan JR, Prasse KW, Mahaffey EA: *Veterinary laboratory medicine: clinical pathology,* ed 3, Ames, 1994, Iowa State University Press.

3. Smith B: *Large animal internal medicine,* St. Louis, 1990, Mosby.

4. Sojka J: Hypothyroidism in horses, *Compend Contin Ed Pract Vet* 17:845-852, 1995.

5. Murray MJ, Luba NK: Plasma gastrin and somatostatin, serum thyroxine (T_4), triiodothyronine (T_3), reverse triodothyronine (rT_3) and cortisol concentrations in foals from birth to 28 days of age, *Equine Vet J* 25:237-239, 1993.

6. Shaftoe S, Schick MP, Chen CL: Thyroid-stimulating hormone response tests in one-day-old foals, *Equine Vet Sci* 8:310-312, 1988.

7. Robinson NE: *Current therapy in equine medicine 2,* Philadelphia, 1987, WB Saunders.

8. Eiler H, Oliver J, Cable D: Adrenal gland function in the horse: effect of dexamethasome on hydrocortisone secretion and blood cellularity and plasma electrolyte concentrations, *Am J Vet Res* 40:727-730, 1979.

9. Colahan PT, Mayhew IA, Merritt AM, Moore JN: *Equine medicine and surgery,* ed 4, Goleta, California, 1991, American Veterinary Publications.

10. Kobluk CN, Ames TR, Leon RJ: *The horse-diseases and clinical management,* Philadelphia, 1995, WB Saunders.

11. Love S: Recognizing disease associated with strongyles in horses, *Compend Contin Ed Pract Vet* 17:564-567, 1995.

12. Uhlinger C: Effects of three anthelmintic schedules on the incidence of colic in horses, *Equine Vet J* 22:251-254, 1990.

13. Mair TS: Recurrent diarrhea in aged ponies associated with larval cyathostomiasis, *Equine Vet J* 25:161-163, 1993.

14. Love S, Mair TS, Hillyer M: Chronic diarrhea in adult horses: a review of 51 referred cases, *Vet Res* 130:217-219, 1992.

15. Cohen ND, Chaffin MK: Causes of diarrhea and enteritis in foals. *Compend Contin Ed Pract Vet* 17:568-574, 1995.

16. Ellis GR, Daniels E: Comparison of direct electron microscopy and enzyme immunoassay for the detection of rotavirus in calves, lambs, piglets, and foals, *Aust Vet J* 65:133-135, 1988.

17. Dwyer RM: Rotaviral diarrhea outbreaks in foals: recommended controls and management, *Vet Med* 86:198-202, 1991.

18. Taylor WM, Bryant JE, Anderson JB, Willers KH: Equine piroplasmosis in the United States: a review, *J Am Vet Med Assoc* 155:915-923, 1969.

19. Holbrook AA: Biology of equine piroplasmosis, *J Am Vet Med Assoc* 155:453-466, 1969.

20. Burgess EC, Mattison M: Encephalitis associated with *Borrelia burgdorferi* infection in a horse, *J Am Vet Med Assoc* 191: 1457-1458, 1987.

21. Madigan JE, Tertler J: Lyme disease in domestic animals, *Proc Am Coll Vet Int Med* 7:811-817, 1989.

22. Magnarelli LA, Anderson JF, Shaw G, Post JE, Palker PC: Borreliosis in equids in northeastern United States, *J Am Vet Med Assoc* 49: 359-362, 1988.

23. Parker JL, White KK: Lyme borreliosis in cattle and horses: a review of the literature, *Cornell Vet* 82:253-274, 1992.

24. Calisher CH, Mahmud Mia, Kafrawi AO, et al: Rapid and specific sero-diagnosis of western equine encephalitis virus infection in horses, *Am J Vet Res* 47:1296-1301, 1986.

25. Keane DP, Little PB, Wilkie BN: Agents of equine viral encephalomyelitis: correlation of serum and cerebrospinal fluid antibodies, *Can J Vet Res* 52:229-233, 1988.

26. Wilson, JH: Strategies for prevention of eastern equine encephalomyelitis, *Proc Am Coll Vet Int Med* 9:423-427, 1991.

27. Madigan JE, Gribble DH: Equine ehrlichiosis in northern California: 49 cases (1968-1981), *J Am Vet Med Assoc* 190:445-452, 1987.

28. Gribble, DH: Equine ehrlichiosis, *J Am Vet Med Assoc* 155:462-470, 1969.

29. Blythe LL, Mattson DE, Lassen ED, Craig AM: Antibodies against equine herpesvirus 1 in the cerebrospinal fluid in the horse, *Can Vet J* 26:218-222, 1985.

30. Clabough DL: Equine infectious anemia: the clinical signs, transmission, and diagnostic procedures, *Vet Med* 85:1007-1113, 1990.

31. Moore BR, Granstrom DG, Reed SM: Diagnosis of equine protozoal myeloencephalitis and cervical stenotic myelopathy. *Compend Contin*

Ed Pract Vet 17:419-426, 1995.

32. Reed SM, Granstrom DE: Equine protozoal encephalomyelitis, *Proc ACVIM Forum* 11:591-592, 1993.

33. Granstrom DE: Diagnosis of equine protozoal myeloencephalitis: Western blot analysis, *Proc Am Coll Vet Int Med* 2:587-590, 1993.

34. Morris DD, Divers TS, Whitlock RH: Renal clearance and fractional excretion of electrolytes over a 24-hour period in horses, *Am J Vet Res* 45:2431-2436, 1984.

35. Kohn CW, Strasser SL: 24-hour renal clearance and excretion of endogenous substances in the mare, *Am J Vet Res* 47:1332-1336, 1986.

36. Bayly WM, Brobst DF, Elfers RS, Reed SM: Serum and urinary biochemistry and enzyme changes in ponies with acute renal failure, *Cornell Vet* 76:306-311, 1986.

37. Andrews FM: Differentiating neurologic diseases in the horse using albumin quotient and IgG index determination, *Am Coll Vet Int Med* 13:600-603, 1995.

38. Brewer BD: Disorders of equine calcium metabolism, *Compend Cont Ed Pract Vet* 4:S244-S250, 1982.

39. Divers TJ, Whitlock RH: Acute renal failure in six horses resulting from haemodynamic causes, *Equine Vet J* 19:178-184, 1987.

40. Moore JN, Steiss J, Nicholson, Orth DN: A case of pituitary adrenocorticotropin-dependent Cushing's syndrome in the horse, *Endocrinology* 104:576-582, 1979.

41. Naylor JM, Robinson JA, Bertone J: Familial incidence of hyperkalemic periodic paralysis in quarter horses, *J Am Vet Med Assoc* 200:340-343, 1992.

42. Richardson DW, Kohn CW: Uroperitoneum in the foal, *J Am Vet Med Assoc* 182:267-271.

43. Shawley RV, Rolf LL Jr: Experimental cantharidiasis in the horse, *Am J Vet Res* 45:2261-2266, 1984.

44. Tennant B, Bettleheim P, Kaneko JJ: Paradoxical hypercalcemia and hypophosphatemia associated with chronic renal failure in horses, *J Am Vet Med Assoc* 180:630-634, 1982.

45. Kaneko JJ: Clinical biochemistry of domestic animals, ed 4, San Diego, 1989, Academic Press.

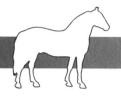

Interpretation of Laboratory Abnormalities

Anemia

Azotemia

Increased GGT

Hyperkalemia

Hypokalemia

Hyponatremia

Metabolic acidosis (adult horses)

The flow diagrams in this section describe an approach to the diagnosis of selected laboratory abnormalities. In some cases, the general causes of the abnormal laboratory test are listed and then followed by appropriate laboratory test results and exam findings used to differentiate these causes. In other diagrams, exam findings or laboratory test results lead to a disease that is discussed in Sections 4 to 14. Discussions for each laboratory test in Section 1 can aid with use and interpretation of these diagrams.

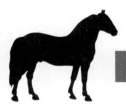

ANEMIA

Anemia is a decrease in red cell number. Anemia is usually classified by response, cell morphology, and cause.

Horses do not release immature red blood cells into circulation during a regenerative response. Therefore, bone marrow cytology is necessary to differentiate regenerative and nonregenerative anemias. Regenerative anemias result in large numbers of erythrocyte precursors in bone marrow smears. If these cells are not present, the anemia is nonregenerative.

Further testing may suggest the cause of the anemia. The appearance of Heinz bodies after new methylene blue staining of blood smears suggests oxidative damage to red blood cells by toxins. Autoagglutination (which must be differentiated from rouleaux by saline dilution) suggests immune-mediated anemia. The presence of antibody on the red blood cell can be confirmed by Coombs testing. Concurrent hypoproteinemia suggests blood loss. Red plasma and hemoglobinuria indicate intravascular hemolysis. Nonregenerative anemias can result from chronic disease or rarely iron deficiency. A low serum iron with a high total iron-binding capacity is consistent with iron deficiency, which occurs rarely with chronic blood loss in horses. A low serum iron with a low total iron-binding capacity is consistent with chronic disease.

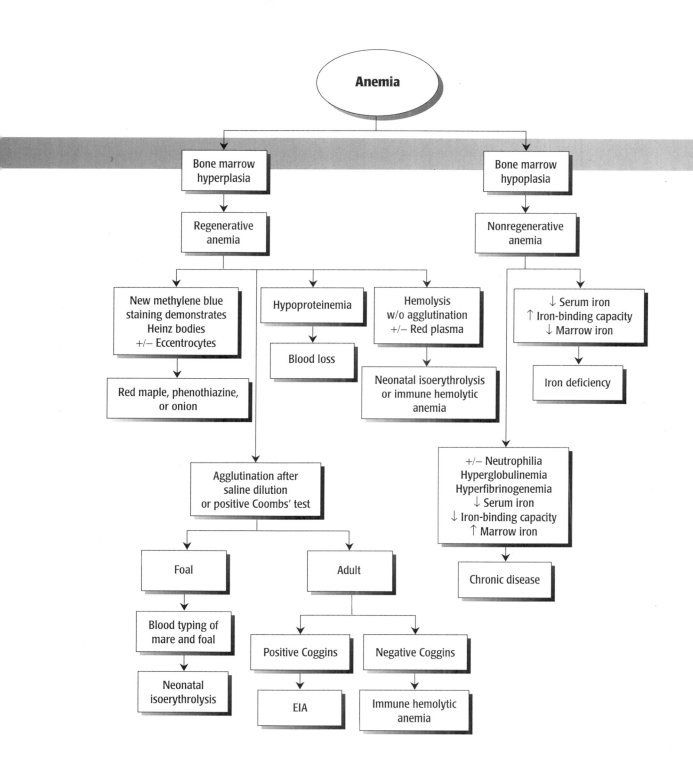

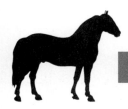

AZOTEMIA

Excess serum urea nitrogen (SUN) or other nitrogenous products constitutes azotemia. Azotemia may occur with renal, prerenal, or postrenal disease.

With increasing failure of the nephron function, there is a decline in the filtration rate of the kidney and an accumulation of urea in the serum, resulting in azotemia. Azotemia of primary renal disease may occur with acute or chronic renal failure. Urine specific gravity is isosthenuric (1.008 to 1.012).

A decrease in renal blood flow without functional change in the kidney, such as dehydration, may cause prerenal azotemia. Urine specific gravity will be concentrated to ⩾1.020.

Postrenal azotemia is usually precipitated by urinary outflow obstruction or rupture of the urinary bladder. Increases of SUN may also be observed with the increased protein catabolism associated with gastrointestinal bleeding or may be caused by diet.

Creatinine is generally considered to be less affected by diet or postrenal resorption than is SUN; however, the creatinine pool is influenced by muscle mass, which may be altered by muscle disease, generalized wasting, and training. Well-muscled animals, such as stallions and draft breeds, have creatinine concentrations in the upper reference range.

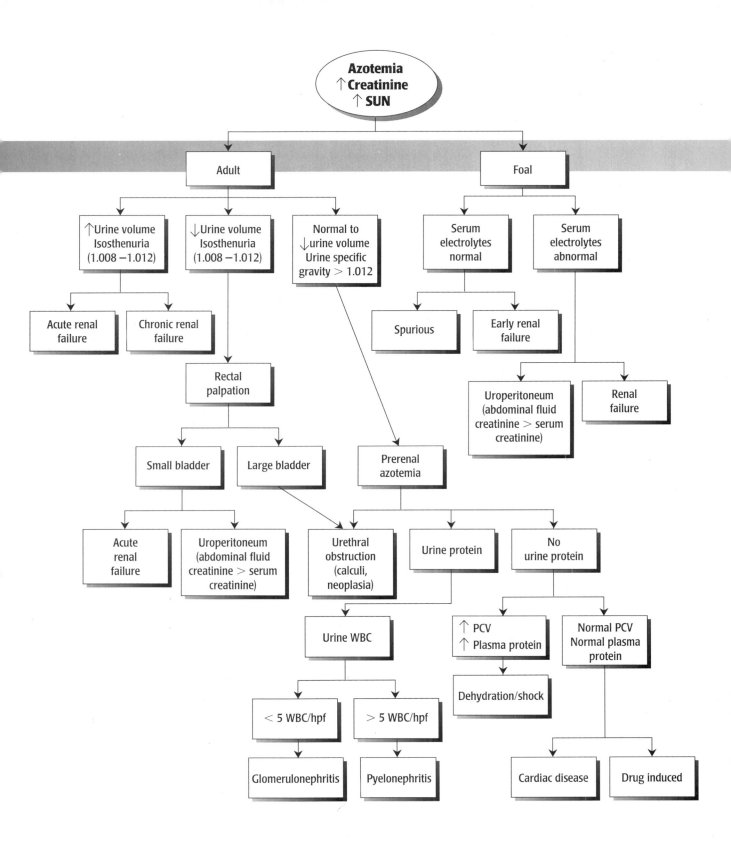

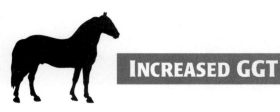

INCREASED GGT

Increases in serum GGT activity are primarily indicative of cholestatic liver disease, but may result from colonic displacement or administration of drugs.

Intrahepatic or extrahepatic cholestasis causes induction of GGT. Intrahepatic cholestasis usually presents with marked increases in SDH and AST activities. SDH and AST activities may be mildly increased with extrahepatic cholestasis. Sonography may reveal dilated canaliculi in extrahepatic cholestasis. A liver biopsy specimen (culture and histology) may be helpful in identifying hepatic disease causing intrahepatic cholestasis.

Increased GGT activity may be detected with obstructive diseases of the large intestine. Induction of GGT activity has been associated with administration of dexamethasone, rifampin, prednisone, and benzimidazole anthelmintics.

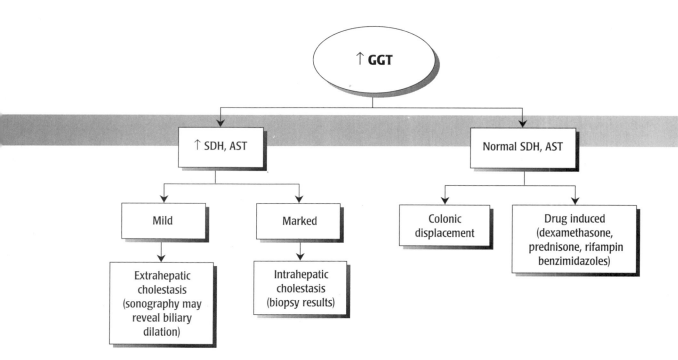

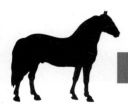

HYPERKALEMIA

Serum potassium is maintained within narrow limits for normal neuro-muscular and cardiac function. Hyperkalemia can lead to life-threatening cardiac conduction abnormalities, bradycardia, and ECG changes.

Hyperkalemia resulting from retention may occur secondary to uroperitoneum, anuric renal failure, or adrenal insufficiency. Azotemia accompanies uroperitoneum and may be differentiated from the azotemia of renal failure by the attendant abdominal distention and high creatinine concentration in the peritoneal fluid. Adrenal insufficiency does not cause abdominal distention or azotemia.

Redistribution from the intracellular compartment to the extracellular compartment causes increased serum potassium. Hyperkalemia may occur in acidemic horses because intracellular potassium exchanges with excess extracellular hydrogen ions. Hyperkalemia occurs during episodes of paralysis in hereditary periodic hyperkalemia and resolves as the episode ends. Insulin deficiency accompanying diabetes results in poor intracellular potassium movement and therefore hyperkalemia.

Because potassium concentration in equine erythrocytes is higher than in plasma, pseudohyperkalemia may rarely occur with marked hemolysis.

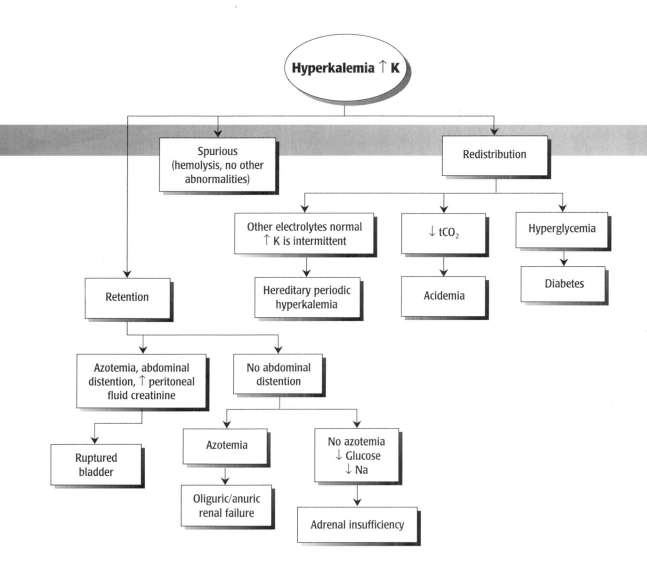

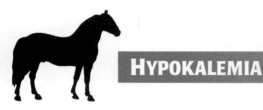

HYPOKALEMIA

Hypokalemia is usually associated with depletion of intracellular stores. Clinical findings include cardiac abnormalities, weakness, and loss of renal concentrating ability.

Anorectic animals develop a negative potassium balance. Loss of gastric and intestinal fluids, which are rich in potassium, produces potassium depletion, such as in diarrhea or choke. Choke is usually diagnosed on the basis of clinical signs of esophageal obstruction. Urinary loss of potassium occurs from the diuresis of polyuria, diuretic therapy, or renal tubular acidosis. Potassium concentration may be normal or decreased in the syndrome of inappropriate ADH. Metabolic alkalemia produces a mild hypokalemia.

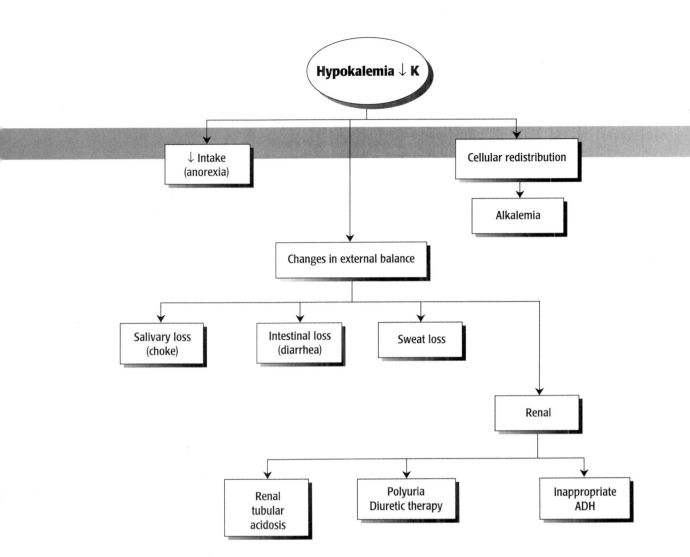

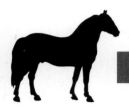

HYPONATREMIA

It is important to evaluate clinical signs, complete electrolyte profiles, and other available laboratory data for proper differential assessment of sodium concentration.

Hyponatremia with hyperkalemia accompanies uroperitoneum and adrenal insufficiency. In animals with uroperitoneum, the large volume of dilute urine that is low in sodium and chloride and high in potassium equilibrates across the large surface area of the peritoneum. Hyponatremia of adrenal insufficiency in horses presents with hyperkalemia, hypoglycemia, hypochloridemia, and sometimes hypocortisolemia.

Diarrhea, excessive sweat and salivary losses, and renal disease can cause hypotonic dehydration (hypovolemia), resulting in characteristic sodium loss with normal and decreased serum potassium. Inappropriate release of antidiuretic hormone, and the dilutional effect of sequestered fluid, such as in edema and ascites, can result in increased total body water and hyponatremia. Treating volume-depleted horses with low-sodium fluids or allowing them to drink electrolyte-free water can create a similar hyponatremia, which may progress from normovolemia to increased total body water.

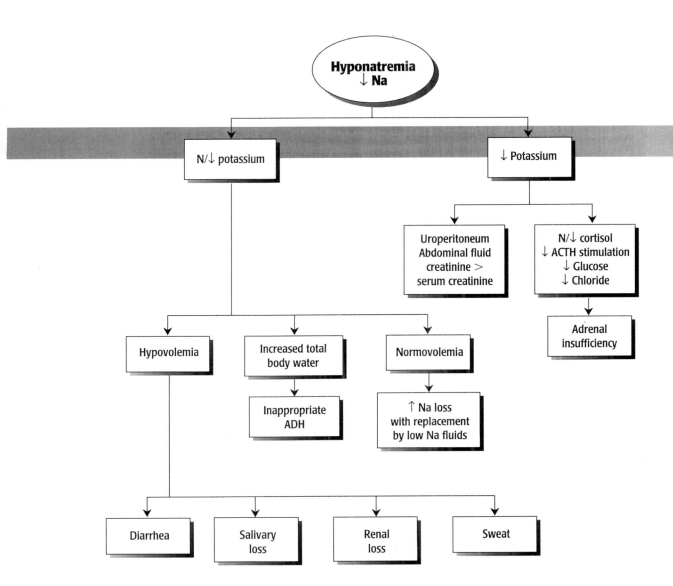

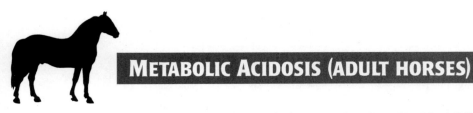

METABOLIC ACIDOSIS (ADULT HORSES)

A decrease in serum total carbon dioxide (tCO_2) indicates metabolic acidosis. Assessment of clinical signs and other laboratory data is necessary to identify the cause of metabolic acidosis.

Lactic acidosis develops in animals with clinical signs of dehydration, as occurs with hypovolemic or endotoxic shock, and cardiac failure causing poor perfusion. Acidosis persisting after rehydration is seen with renal disease and colitis. Renal failure and the ensuing accumulation of uremic acids can cause a titrational metabolic acidosis. Bicarbonate loss in intestinal disease with diarrhea and in renal tubular acidosis with bicarbonate loss results in metabolic acidosis. A secondary compensatory metabolic acidosis should occur with respiratory alkalosis associated with pulmonary diseases, such as hypotension, pulmonary vascular shunts, pulmonary fibrosis, pneumonia, and pulmonary edema.

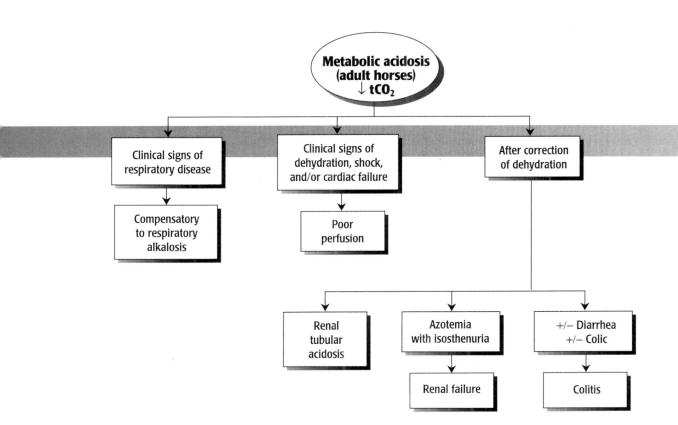

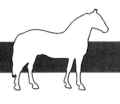

Clinical Signs

Acute diarrhea

Cardiac dysrhythmias

Chronic diarrhea

Coughing

Dysuria

Edema

Epistaxis

Fever

Icterus

Muscular pain, rigidity, or spasm

Pigmenturia

Seizures

Weakness

Weight loss

The flow diagrams in this section describe an approach to diagnosis based on abnormal clinical signs. In some cases, the general causes of the abnormal clinical signs are listed and then followed by laboratory test results and exam findings used to differentiate these causes. In other diagrams, clinical findings or laboratory test results lead to a disease that is discussed in Sections 4 to 14. Discussions for each laboratory test in Section 1 can aid with use and interpretation of these diagrams. Selected laboratory results are indicated for some diseases. Sections 4 to 14 must be consulted for a more complete list of laboratory results.

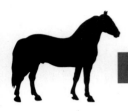

ACUTE DIARRHEA

Intestinal obstruction, peritonitis, enterocolitis, dietary alterations, and liver failure are potential causes of acute diarrhea. Laboratory assessment alone is generally inadequate for differentiation of acute diarrhea and must be used in conjunction with all other assessment techniques.

Acute peritonitis sometimes results in either endotoxemia or sequestration of neutrophils in the abdominal cavity such that neutropenia and a left shift occur. Increased abdominal fluid cell count and protein concentration confirm the presence of peritonitis.

Endotoxemia and intestinal inflammation commonly result in neutropenia and a left shift in horses with enterocolitis. Hyponatremia, hypokalemia, hypochloridemia, and decreased total CO_2 are common abnormalities in horses with acute secretory diarrhea, especially when it is caused by salmonellosis. Further assessment of the cause of enterocolitis requires other testing procedures.

Liver failure can be confirmed by increased bilirubin and prolonged BSP clearance. Hypoglycemia and abnormal clotting times also commonly result from liver failure. Serum concentrations of liver enzymes (SDH, AST, GGT) and bile acids are commonly elevated in liver disease.

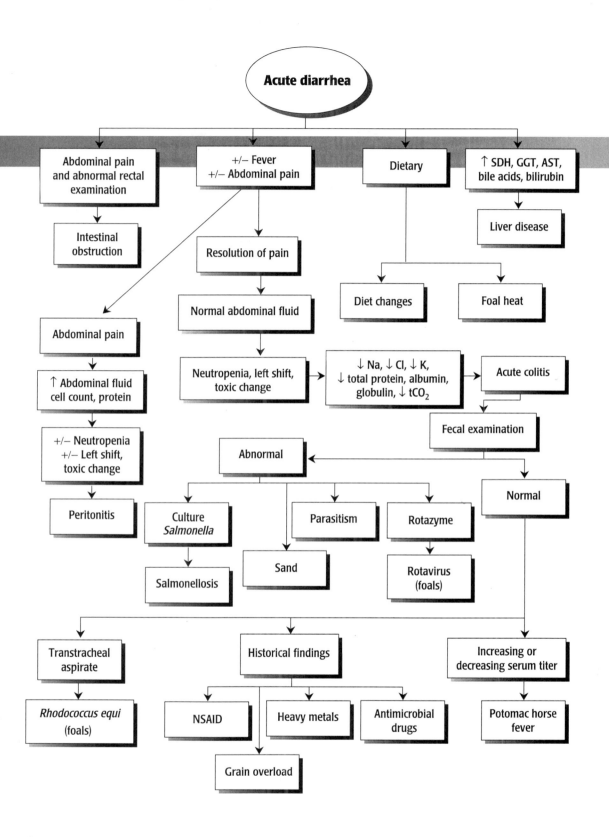

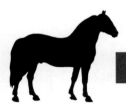

CARDIAC DYSRHYTHMIAS

Cardiac dysrhythmias may cause syncope, exercise intolerance, or death. Cardiac rhythm disturbances can result from metabolic abnormalities or from cardiac disease. Laboratory evaluation is helpful for the assessment of metabolic factors; however, other techniques allow more complete assessment of cardiac function. Electrocardiography is necessary in all cases to evaluate the type of dysrhythmia.

Electrolyte abnormalities are among the most common causes of cardiac dysrhythmias and are easily evaluated with laboratory testing. Toxemia resulting from endotoxemia or bacterial infection is sometimes accompanied by neutropenia, left shift, and toxic changes. Hypoxia and increased PCO_2 can develop in association with respiratory disease, cardiovascular disease, or anesthesia.

Specific cardiac abnormalities include myocarditis, cardiomyopathy, congenital defects, valvular defects, or pericardial disease. Active damage to myocardial cells (myocarditis or cardiomyopathy) is frequently accompanied by elevations in the serum concentration of cardiac fractions of CK (CKMB) isoenzymes. Other cardiac abnormalities are assessed via echocardiography.

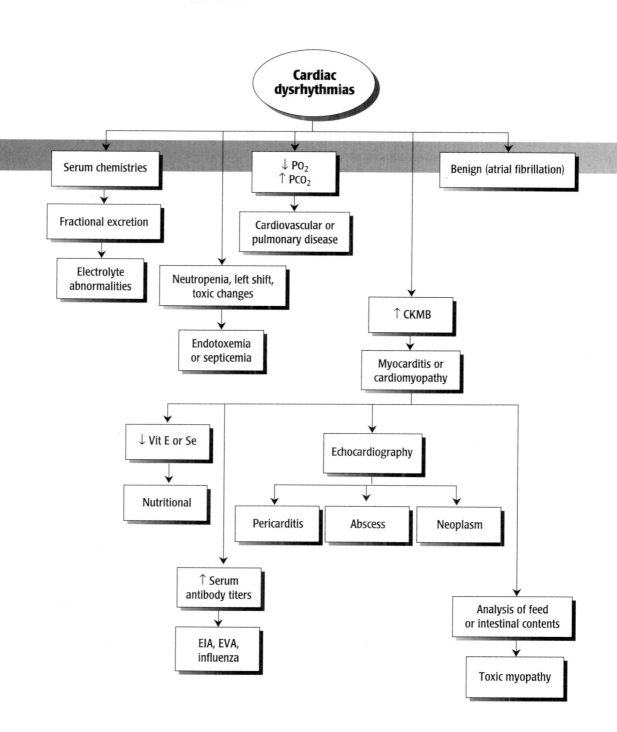

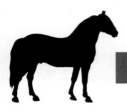

CHRONIC DIARRHEA

Diarrhea is frequent passage of unformed feces. The condition is chronic when it is present for more than 1 month. Diet, gastrointestinal disease, and systemic disease can all result in chronic diarrhea. Weight loss commonly accompanies gastrointestinal and systemic disease.

Many dietary factors can cause diarrhea, and not all are readily apparent by examination of the diet. Diets that are high in digestible carbohydrate and poor-quality roughage are some of the more common causes of chronic diarrhea. Less obvious dietary causes only become evident after there is a positive response to diet changes.

Liver disease and cardiac disease can sometimes result in chronic diarrhea. Liver disease is accompanied by increases in the serum activity of GGT, SDH, and AST. Increased serum concentration of bilirubin and bile acids occurs when there is liver failure. Heart failure is best evaluated by other methods, including physical examination and echocardiography.

Gastrointestinal diseases are the most common causes of chronic diarrhea. Abdominal abscessation, granulomatous enteritis, and lymphosarcoma can all affect the small intestine, causing malabsorption of important nutrients, glucose, and xylose. These diseases are also sometimes accompanied by changes in serum protein concentration. Abdominal abscessation is associated with septic inflammation, which increases the plasma fibrinogen concentration, plasma globulin concentration, and abdominal fluid cell count and causes nonregenerative anemia. Lymphosarcoma often causes a polyclonal gammopathy; however, it is occasionally associated with a monoclonal gammopathy. Granulomatous enteritis is almost always accompanied by intestinal protein loss. Diagnosis of lymphosarcoma and granulomatous enteritis is dependent on intestinal biopsy. Salmonellosis, sand-induced colitis, and NSAID toxicity cause more colonic damage than small intestinal damage. Therefore, diarrhea usually occurs without malabsorption of glucose or xylose. Intestinal protein loss is variable with these diseases. Diagnosis of these conditions is based on fecal culture and examination and history of drug administration.

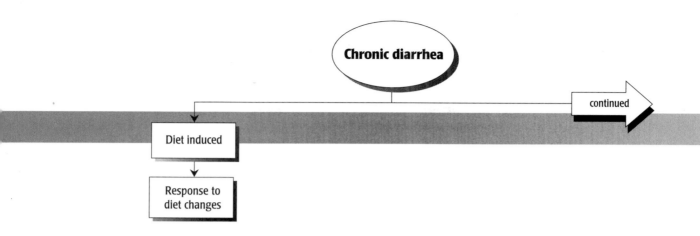

Chronic diarrhea

Diet induced

Response to
diet changes

continued

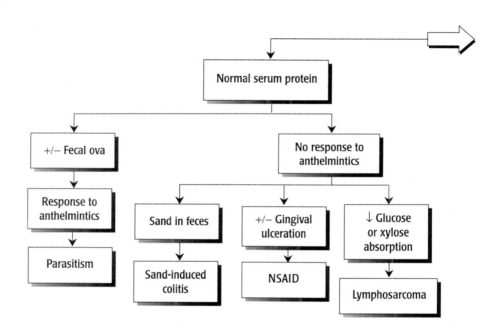

Normal serum protein

+/– Fecal ova

Response to
anthelmintics

Parasitism

No response to
anthelmintics

Sand in feces

Sand-induced
colitis

+/– Gingival
ulceration

NSAID

↓ Glucose
or xylose
absorption

Lymphosarcoma

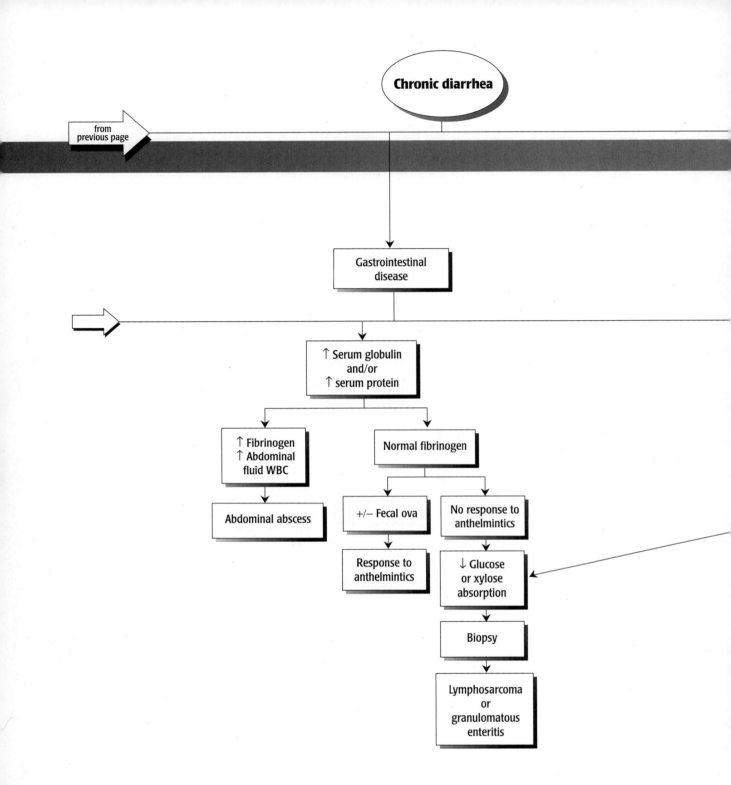

Chronic diarrhea

from previous page

Gastrointestinal
disease

↑ Serum globulin
and/or
↑ serum protein

↑ Fibrinogen
↑ Abdominal
fluid WBC

Normal fibrinogen

Abdominal abscess

+/− Fecal ova

No response to
anthelmintics

Response to
anthelmintics

↓ Glucose
or xylose
absorption

Biopsy

Lymphosarcoma
or
granulomatous
enteritis

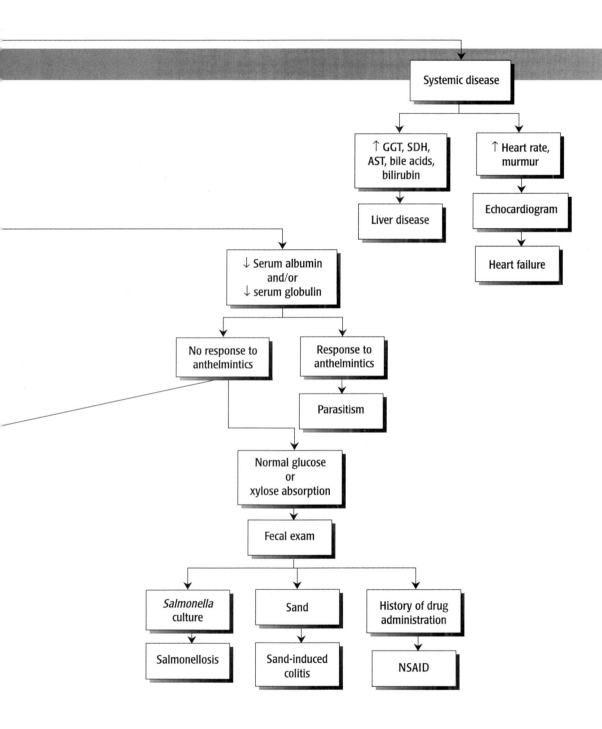

Systemic disease

↑ GGT, SDH, AST, bile acids, bilirubin → Liver disease

↑ Heart rate, murmur → Echocardiogram → Heart failure

↓ Serum albumin and/or ↓ serum globulin

No response to anthelmintics

Response to anthelmintics → Parasitism

Normal glucose or xylose absorption → Fecal exam

Salmonella culture → Salmonellosis

Sand → Sand-induced colitis

History of drug administration → NSAID

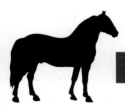

COUGHING

Coughing can result from upper respiratory or pulmonary disease. When accompanied by fever, neutrophilia, and increased plasma fibrinogen concentration, bacterial diseases such as pneumonia and *Streptococcus equi* infection are commonly diagnosed. Viral respiratory diseases often result in fever without changes in white blood cell count and plasma fibrinogen concentration.

Numerous upper respiratory diseases can cause coughing without causing concurrent fever. These are better evaluated by methods other than laboratory testing. Bacterial bronchitis and chronic obstructive pulmonary disease are lower respiratory tract diseases that can cause coughing without fever. These are evaluated with thoracic radiography and transtracheal aspiration.

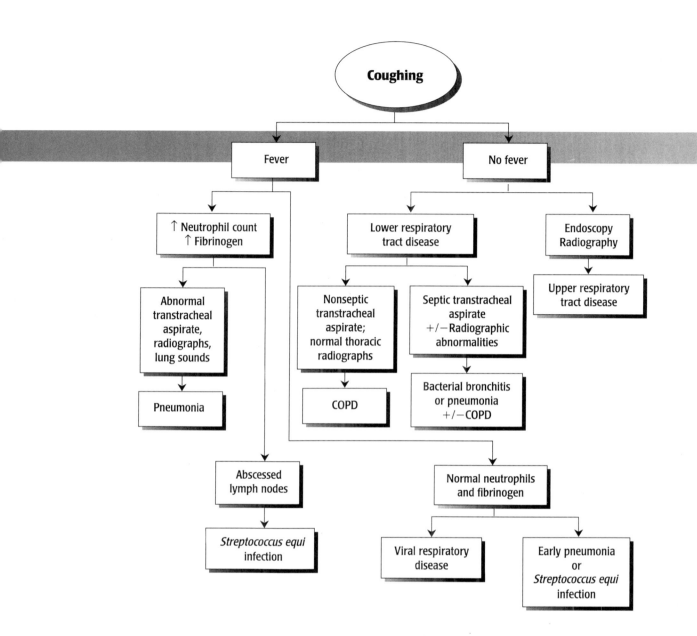

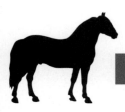

DYSURIA

Cystitis, urinary calculi, neoplasia, and neurologic abnormalities involving sacral and coccygeal nerves can result in urinary incontinence. Cystitis increases the red blood cell count (hematuria), neutrophil count (pyuria), and protein (proteinuria) in urine. Occult blood testing on dipstick is frequently positive because of hemolysis of the blood in the urine before processing of the sample. Cystic calculi and neoplasia commonly result in hematuria. Calculi, neoplastic diseases, and neurologic abnormalities often result in cystitis and, therefore, pyuria.

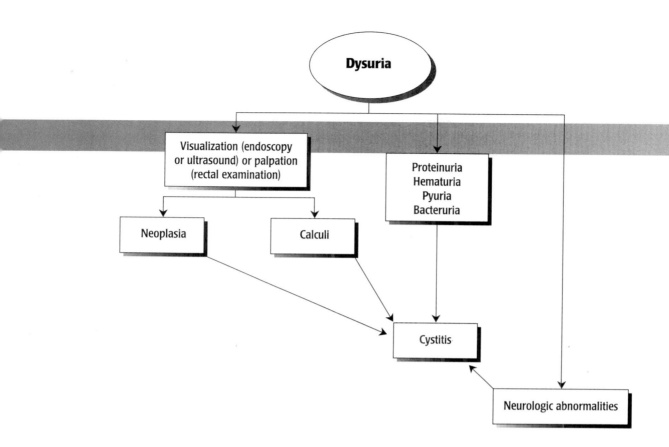

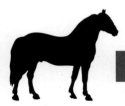

EDEMA

Edema is abnormal accumulation of extracellular fluid resulting from increased hydrostatic pressure, decreased plasma oncotic pressure, increased capillary permeability, and decreased lymphatic flow. Neoplasia or abscessation can result in edema caused by increased capillary hydrostatic pressure or decreased lymphatic flow. Specific diagnosis of these problems is based on cytology, culture, or biopsy (neoplasia). Heart failure leads to increased capillary hydrostatic pressure and is evaluated via echocardiography and electrocardiography. Vasculitis is suspected when there are edema and petechiation with a normal platelet count; it is confirmed with a skin biopsy.

Laboratory evaluation is most useful in evaluation of hypoproteinemia and/or hypoalbuminemia as a cause of edema. Causes of hypoproteinemia include decreased protein production (starvation and liver failure) and increased protein loss (protein-losing enteropathy or glomerulopathy).

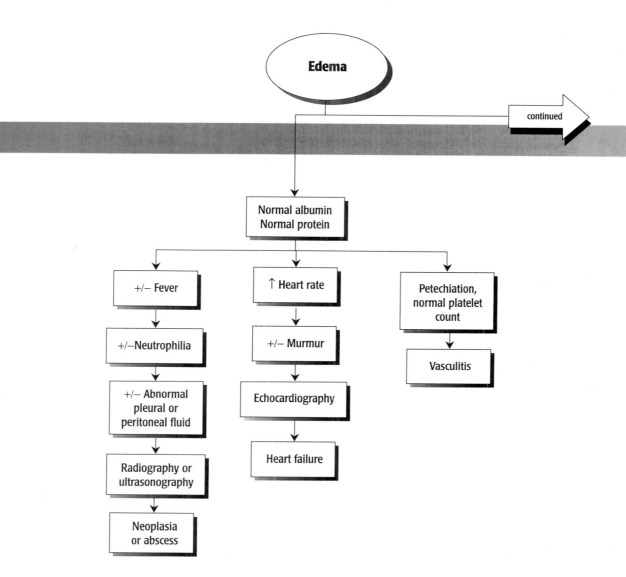

continued

Edema

Normal albumin
Normal protein

+/− Fever

+/−Neutrophilia

+/− Abnormal
pleural or
peritoneal fluid

Radiography or
ultrasonography

Neoplasia
or abscess

↑ Heart rate

+/− Murmur

Echocardiography

Heart failure

Petechiation,
normal platelet
count

Vasculitis

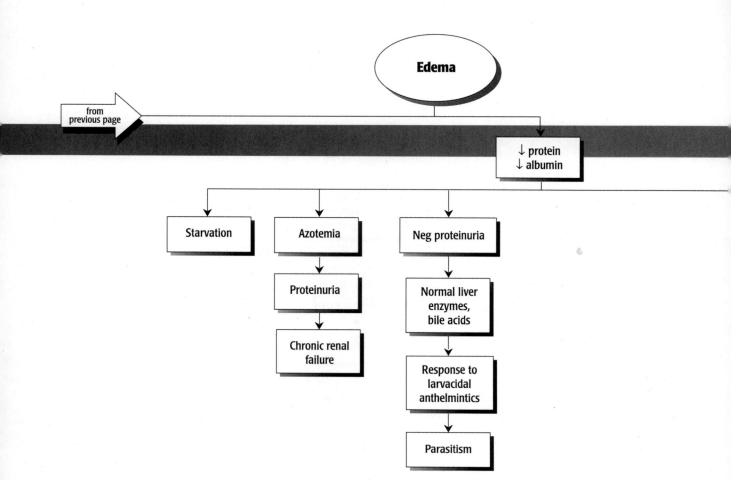

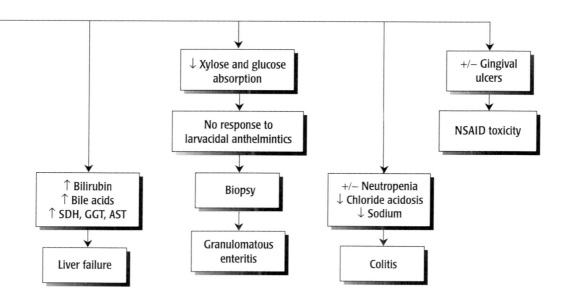

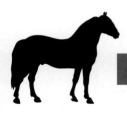

EPISTAXIS

Nasal discharge of blood results from clotting abnormalities, upper respiratory tract hemorrhage, or lower respiratory tract hemorrhage. Thrombocytopenia, which can be confirmed by quantitation of platelet numbers, can lead to epistaxis in horses with disseminated intravascular coagulation (DIC) or immune-mediated thrombocytopenia. DIC is often accompanied by increased concentration of fibrinogen degradation products and prolongation of clotting times.

Decreased concentrations of clotting factors result in prolongation of clotting times (APTT and OSPT) without changes in platelet number. Liver failure, a common cause of clotting factor abnormalities, is diagnosed by elevations in serum enzyme activities (GGT, SDH, AST), bilirubin, and bile acids. Warfarin toxicity and moldy sweet clover are usually diagnosed by history and confirmation of normal liver function. However, special laboratory testing can allow assay of coumarins in the serum.

Respiratory tract lesions resulting in epistaxis are best assessed by techniques other than laboratory testing.

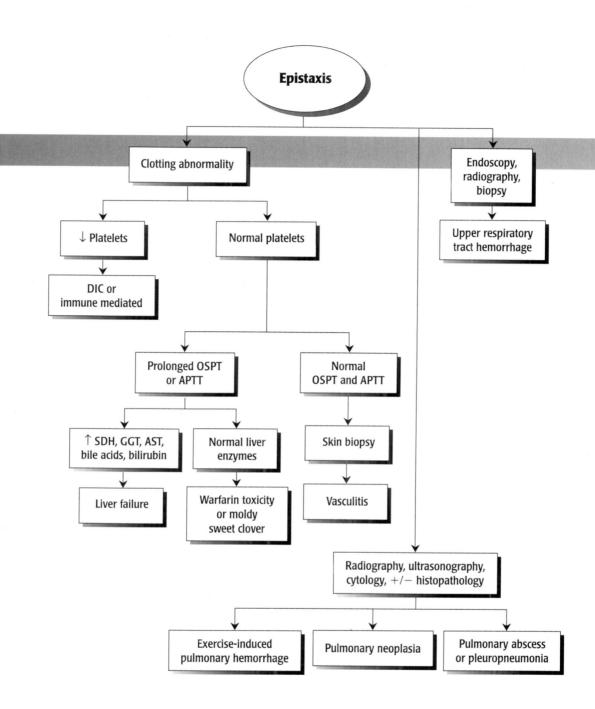

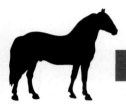

FEVER

Fever is a common clinical sign associated with numerous disease processes. Laboratory testing can be used as an initial assessment of the source of fever. However, the results of laboratory tests are not consistent and should not be used alone to definitively rule in or out any of these diseases.

Colitis, peritonitis, and other inflammatory processes resulting in endotoxemia commonly cause margination of neutrophils and neutropenia. Tissue inflammation stimulates neutrophils to leave the vascular space. With massive acute inflammation tissue sequestration can exceed the rate of release from the bone marrow, thereby decreasing the circulating neutrophil count. Band neutrophils and neutrophils with toxic changes are commonly released from the bone marrow (left shift) under these conditions. Viral diseases and those diseases causing mild inflammation (neoplastic diseases) may be accompanied by no change in the complete blood count. Chronic septic inflammation and neoplastic diseases will stimulate release of mature neutrophils from the bone marrow, causing increases in the number of circulating neutrophils. These chronic conditions are commonly accompanied by an increase in the plasma fibrinogen and serum globulin concentrations and a nonregenerative anemia.

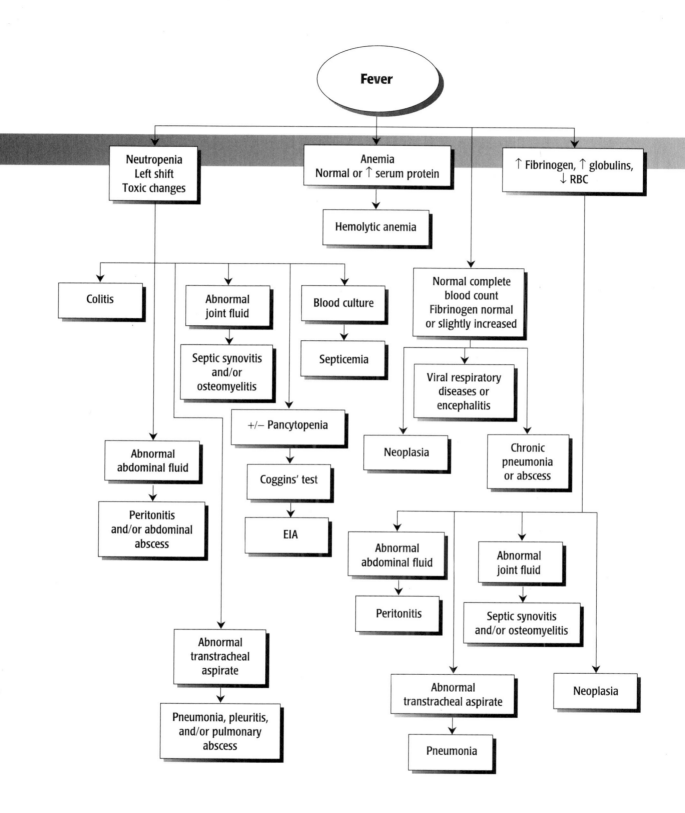

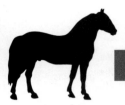

ICTERUS

Icterus is yellow discoloration of the mucous membranes and sclera owing to increased amounts of bilirubin in tissues and serum. Tissues can show yellow discoloration with normal serum bilirubin concentration, owing to dietary pigments. Elevations of total serum bilirubin result from anorexia or systemic disease, liver failure, or hemolytic anemia. Moderate icterus commonly occurs in response to fasting or anorexia. This increase in bilirubin (often up to 10 mg/dl) is almost entirely indirect (unconjugated) bilirubin.

Hemolytic anemia results from intravascular or extravascular destruction of red blood cells. Serum bilirubin concentration often increases, since this destruction results in production of bilirubin more rapidly than can be removed by the liver. The increase in total bilirubin results from an increase in indirect (unconjugated) bilirubin and is accompanied by a decrease in the red blood cell count and packed cell volume. Intravascular hemolysis may also result in hemoglobinuria and hemoglobinemia.

Liver failure impairs uptake and excretion of bilirubin. Both direct (conjugated) and indirect (unconjugated) bilirubin can be increased during liver failure. The direct (conjugated) bilirubin is 15% to 40% of the total bilirubin in horses with liver failure. Active liver damage can increase the serum activity of SDH and AST. Elevations of the serum activity of GGT and AP indicate intrahepatic or extrahepatic cholestasis. Bile acids and BSP clearance testing are abnormal in liver failure.

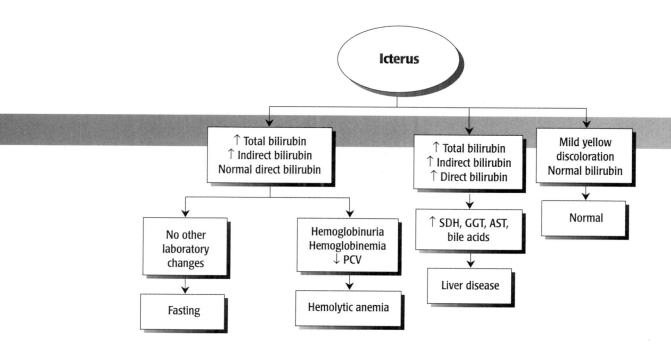

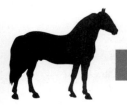

MUSCULAR PAIN, RIGIDITY, OR SPASM

Muscular rigidity or spasm can be caused by abnormalities of the cellular transmembrane potential resulting from electrolyte abnormalities, neurologic disease, or muscular disease. Electrolyte abnormalities are evaluated by measuring the serum concentration or by evaluating the fractional urinary excretion. Periodic hyperkalemic paralysis is associated with normal fractional urinary excretion and intermittent abnormalities of serum potassium concentration. Muscular rigidity is a common sign of hypocalcemia, which can result from the excessive calcium demand created by lactation (lactation tetany), transport tetany, blister beetle toxicosis (plus hypomagnesemia), and exhaustion. Potassium depletion can reduce the intracellular potassium concentration before causing hypokalemia. This can affect muscle function and can be documented by measuring the fractional urinary excretion of potassium.

Neurologic diseases are often accompanied by mild elevations of the serum activity of enzymes found within muscle cells (CK, AST). However, these elevations are usually easily differentiated from the dramatic increases associated with diseases localized to the muscle cell. Submaximal exercise testing can help differentiate muscular disease from other causes of pain when rest has allowed CK and AST to return to normal. Further testing is necessary to differentiate between the specific causes of neurologic or muscular disease.

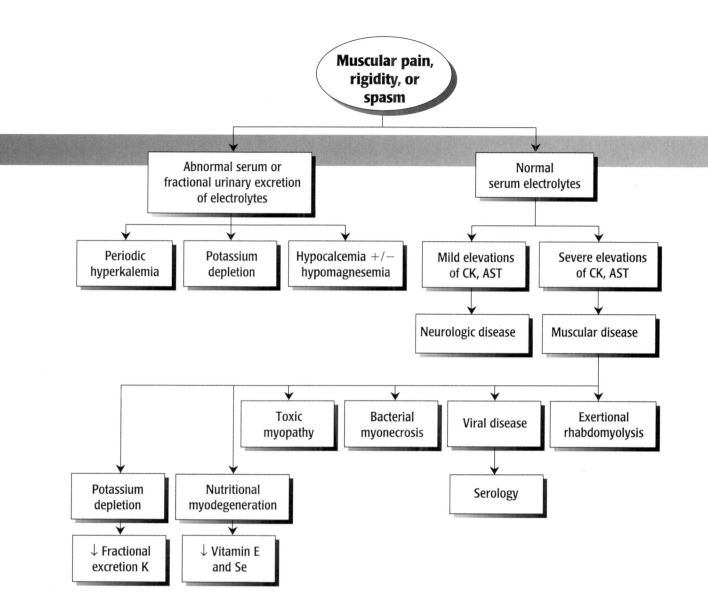

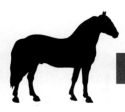

PIGMENTURIA

Hemoglobin and myoglobin cause a red or brown discoloration of the urine and give a positive reaction on urine occult blood dipsticks. Both are potent tubular toxins that can cause azotemia. Hematuria also may discolor the urine, but centrifugation will result in clearing.

Hemoglobinuria results from intravascular hemolysis, which causes a decease in the red blood cell count and a regenerative anemia. Hemoglobin is filtered more slowly by the glomerulus than is myoglobin, and hemoglobinemia sometimes causes red discoloration of the plasma. The presence of hemoglobin in urine may be detected by precipitation with ammonium sulfate.

Myoglobinuria is associated with clinical evidence of muscle damage (usually stiffness and pain). The serum activities of AST and CK are increased. In cases where rest has allowed CK and AST to return to normal, submaximal exercise testing is frequently abnormal. Myoglobin is a smaller molecule, which moves quickly across the glomerular membrane from plasma into the urine without discoloring the plasma.

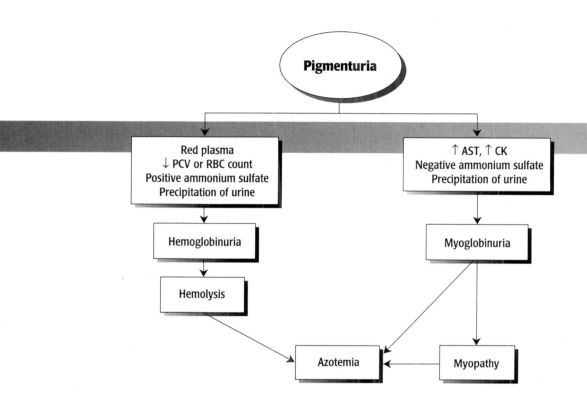

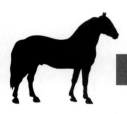

SEIZURES

A seizure is generalized or localized involuntary motor activity resulting from abnormal electrical activity in the brain. Opisthotonos, paddling, and extensor rigidity are common clinical signs. Potential causes include metabolic abnormalities, toxins, neuromuscular diseases, encephalitis, trauma, meningitis, and idiopathic epilepsy.

Hypoxia can be identified by blood gas analysis, and the cardiovascular or respiratory diseases causing hypoxia are best evaluated by nonlaboratory methods. Decreased total CO_2 can result from lactic acid accumulation during poor perfusion or bicarbonate loss from renal or gastrointestinal disease. Liver failure will increase liver enzymes, bile acids, and bilirubin. Hypoglycemia is most common in neonates, but also results from liver failure in adult horses. Electrolyte abnormalities can also lead to seizures.

Meningitis, trauma, encephalitis, neuromuscular diseases, and toxins are evaluated by history, physical examination, antibody titers, CSF cytology, and radiography.

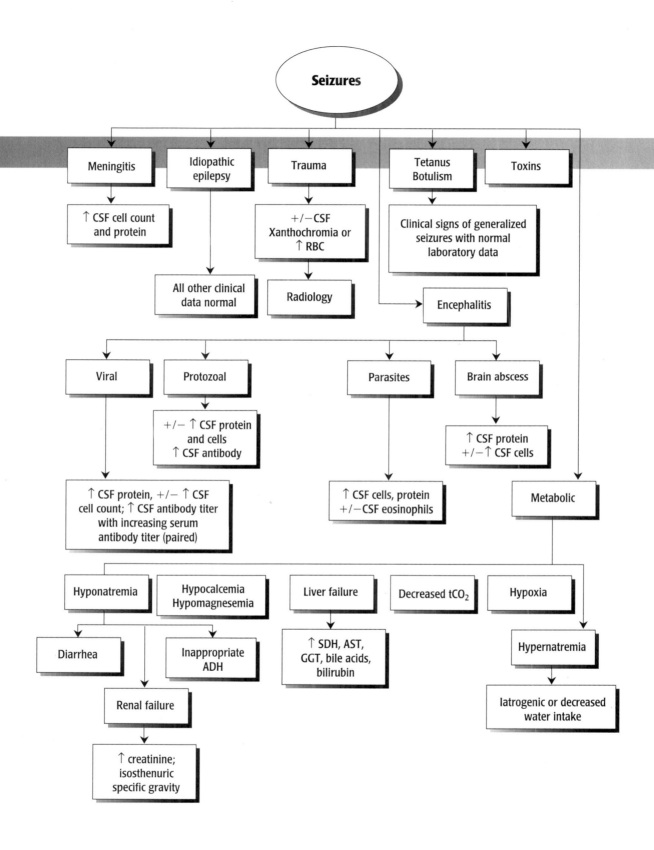

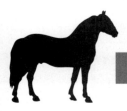

WEAKNESS

Weakness can result from metabolic abnormalities, neurological disease, poor tissue perfusion or oxygenation, and inflammatory disease. Laboratory testing is especially useful in assessment of metabolic diseases. Any disease that decreases feed intake frequently causes hypokalemia, which commonly manifests as depression and muscular weakness. Hyperkalemic periodic paralysis may result in intermittent episodes of hyperkalemia, which can result in weakness. Hyperkalemia occurs rarely in horses with azotemia. Liver failure (which increases SDH, GGT, bilirubin, bile acids) can sometimes cause hypoglycemia. Because neonates have a poor hepatic glycogen reserve, hypoglycemia occurs rapidly when milk intake is inadequate or when concurrent disease (especially sepsis) increases the energy needs. Whenever feed intake is inadequate for energy needs, pregnant pony or miniature horse mares commonly develop hyperlipemia, which can be accompanied by hypoglycemia or liver failure. Inadequate nutrition resulting from starvation or malabsorptive diseases can result in weakness. Prolonged starvation and malabsorption can result in hypoalbuminemia owing to inadequate protein synthesis. Malabsorption can usually be documented by xylose and glucose absorption testing. Organ failure such as in azotemia (increased creatinine) and hepatic failure (increased SDH, GGT, bilirubin, bile acids) are other metabolic causes of weakness.

Poor tissue perfusion can result from hypovolemic or endotoxic shock and cardiac failure. Hypovolemic or endotoxic shock can lead to hemoconcentration, which increases red blood cell count, protein concentration, and creatinine. Endotoxic shock also causes margination of neutrophils, resulting in neutropenia. Cardiac failure is best evaluated by electrocardiography, echocardiography, and physical examination. Hypoxia can be documented by blood gas analysis. The cardiac and pulmonary diseases causing hypoxia are assessed by nonlaboratory techniques.

Mediators of inflammation can also result in weakness. Chronic inflammation can be accompanied by increased concentration of globulins and fibrinogen and depression anemia. Acute inflammation may decrease or increase the white blood cell count and cause increases in fibrinogen concentration (after 48 hours). Diseases causing inflammation are evaluated by other techniques.

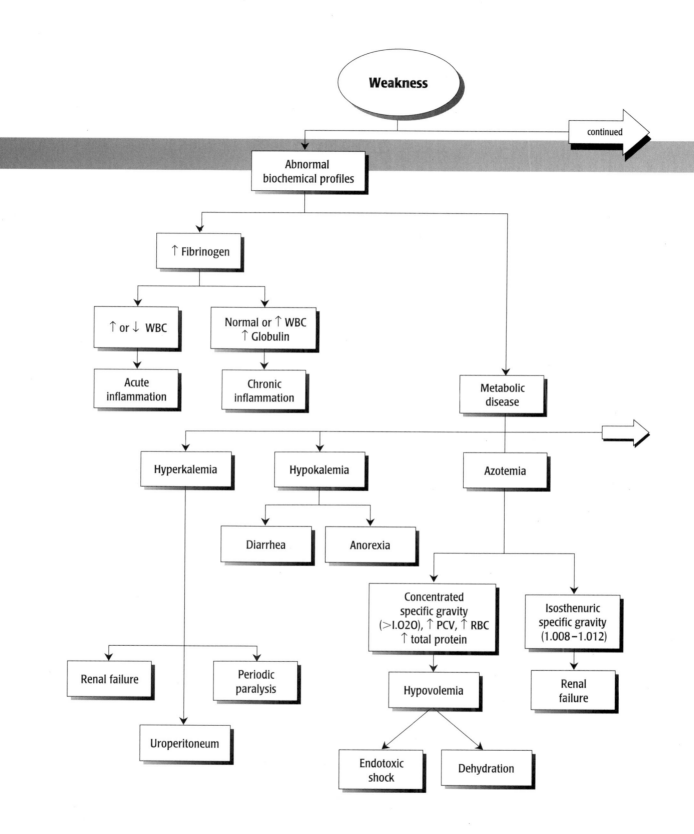

continued

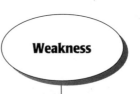

Weakness

from previous page

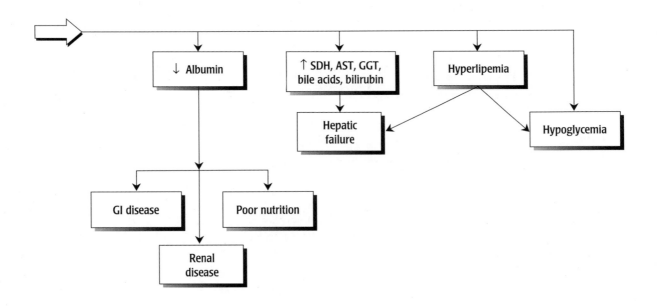

↓ Albumin

↑ SDH, AST, GGT, bile acids, bilirubin

Hyperlipemia

Hepatic failure

Hypoglycemia

GI disease

Poor nutrition

Renal disease

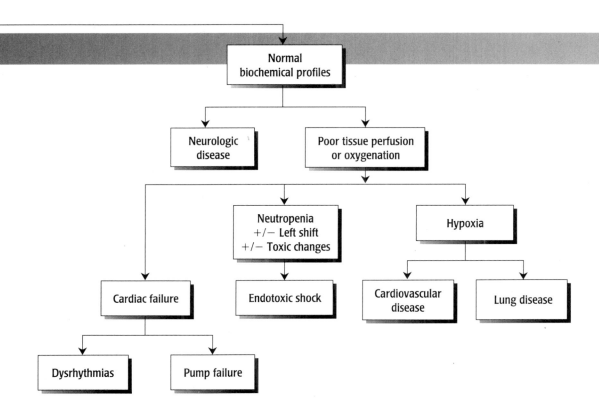

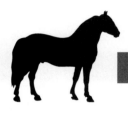

WEIGHT LOSS

Weight loss can result from improper nutrition, inability to masticate feed owing to dental abnormalities, disease processes causing anorexia, and disease processes causing rapid utilization of calories. History and physical examination are used to differentiate dental disease and adequacy of nutrition. Gastrointestinal, renal, endocrine, liver, cardiac, and pulmonary diseases that are of chronic duration can lead to weight loss. A more complicated series of diagnostic tests is necessary to confirm some diseases that affect multiple organ systems (e.g., neoplasia). These diseases are, therefore, not discussed here.

Gastrointestinal diseases are among the most common causing weight loss. Small intestinal disease can result in impaired absorption of glucose and xylose. Gastrointestinal diseases may cause increased (due to inflammation) or decreased (protein-losing enteropathy) serum protein, globulin, or albumin concentration. Parasitism is very common and can be associated with either no laboratory abnormalities, increased serum protein and globulin, or decreased protein and albumin. Because the clinical findings of parasitism overlap with those of many other intestinal diseases, diagnosis is often based on response to larvacidal anthelmintic therapy.

Pituitary adenoma is an endocrine disease resulting in weight loss in horses. Liver, cardiovascular, respiratory, and renal disease can be manifested as chronic weight loss. Azotemia and proteinuria are useful in the diagnosis of chronic renal diseases. Liver disease is usually accompanied by elevation of liver enzymes, bile acids, and bilirubin. Equine infectious anemia (EIA) can be accompanied by anemia, leukopenia, and thrombocytopenia and is confirmed by antibody testing. Respiratory disease causing weight loss is usually pulmonary and is septic (pneumonia) or nonseptic (chronic obstructive pulmonary diseases; COPD). Septic disease can be accompanied by increases in plasma fibrinogen and white blood cell count, whereas horses with COPD have a normal plasma fibrinogen concentration and WBC count.

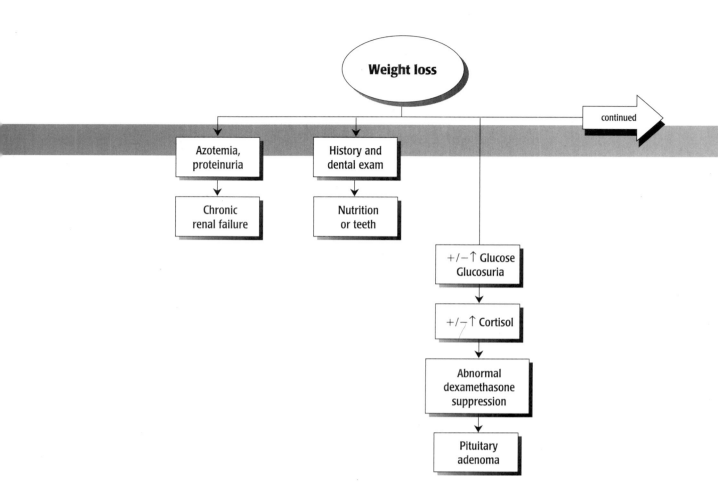

continued

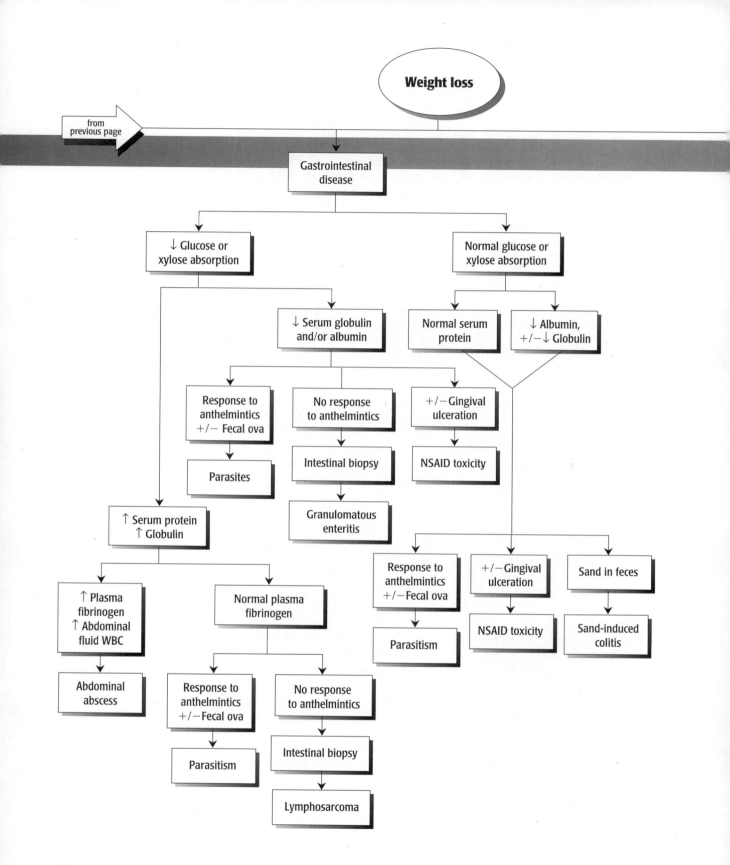

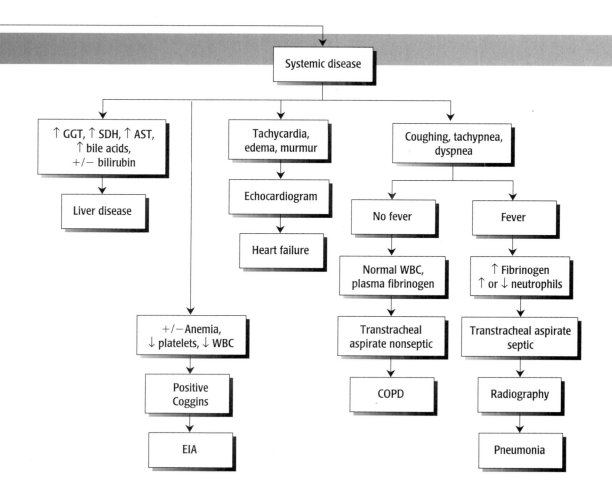

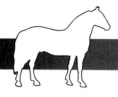

Cardiovascular Diseases

Valvular diseases

Myocarditis and cardiomyopathy

Pericarditis

Congenital cardiovascular disease

Septic thrombophlebitis

Septicemia

Vasculitis

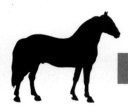

VALVULAR DISEASES

Diseases of the aortic, pulmonic, mitral, and tricuspid valves can lead to valvular dysfunction. Valvular damage usually results in regurgitant flow sometimes progressing to congestive heart failure. Therefore, clinical signs can include a prominent murmur, tachycardia, venous distention, dependent edema, and exercise intolerance. Valvular disease results from either degeneration, bacterial infection, or chordae rupture. Degeneration is a change associated with aging. Chordae rupture can result from valvular disease or can occur idiopathically. Bacterial infection (endocarditis) occurs secondary to transient or sustained bacteremia. Bacterial isolates include streptococci, *Antinobacillus equuli*, and *Escherichia coli*. Ventricular dilation resulting from myocarditis can lead to valvular insufficiency.

INTERPRETATION OF LABORATORY DATA

When valvular damage progresses to congestive heart failure, glomerular filtration is reduced, thereby increasing SUN and creatinine. Hepatic necrosis resulting from congestion may cause elevations in serum activity of AST and SDH. When valvular disease is due to bacterial endocarditis, inflammation and chronic immune stimulation can be indicated by increased plasma fibrinogen and serum globulin concentrations, neutrophilia (with or without a left shift), and a nonregenerative anemia. Septic nephritis and hepatitis resulting from bacterial embolism are uncommon causes of elevations in SUN, creatinine, and serum activity of AST and SDH. When renal failure increases SUN and creatinine, urine specific gravity is in the isosthenuric range. Septic nephritis can increase quantities of blood, protein, WBC, RBC, and bacteria in urine.

SIGNIFICANT DISEASES TO RULE OUT

◆ Myocarditis or cardiomyopathy results in elevation of serum concentrations of enzymes specific to cardiac muscle cells, including CKMB.
◆ Echocardiographic examination of valves is normal.

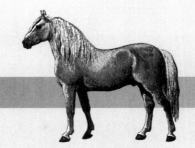

Signs

◆ Murmur
◆ Tachycardia
◆ Venous distention
◆ Edema
◆ Exercise intolerance

Serum Chemistry

	low	normal	high
CK			
AST	.†	.†	
SDH	.†	.†	
GGT			
bile acids			
bilirubin, total			
bilirubin, direct			
protein, total	•	•	
albumin			
globulin	•	•	
SUN	.†	.†	
creatinine	.†	.†	
glucose			
Ca			
P			
Na			
K			
Cl			
tCO₂			

Hemogram

	low	normal	high
total RBC	•	•	
PCV	•	•	
total WBC		•	•
neutrophils		•	•
bands		•	•
lymphocytes			
monocytes			
eosinophils			
basophils			
platelets			
fibrinogen		•	•

Urinalysis

	normal	abnormal
color		
blood	•	•
protein	•	•
albumin		
glucose		
pH		
specific gravity	•	•
WBC	•	•
RBC	•	•
epithelial cells		
bacteria	•	•
casts		
crystals		

Special Tests

◆ Echocardiography may reveal increased ventricular and atrial dimensions, or thickened, shaggy, ragged, fluttering, or prolapsing valves.
◆ Doppler echocardiography may reveal regurgitant flow.
◆ Microbiology may reveal positive blood cultures in cases of vegetative endocarditis.

• Changes caused by the disease itself
•† Changes secondary to dysfunction caused by the disease

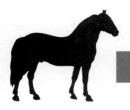

MYOCARDITIS AND CARDIOMYOPATHY

Inflammation of the myocardium can result from either viral disease (equine infectious anemia and equine influenza), bacterial disease, or endotoxemia. Cardiomyopathy refers to obscure diseases of the heart muscle. Cardiomyopathy has been associated with nutritional imbalances (vitamin E and selenium deficiency) and intoxication with monensin, lasalocid, gossypol, and *Cassia* spp. When myocarditis or cardiomyopathy is not severe, clinical signs associated with other organ systems will predominate (e.g., respiratory illness with influenza). With severe myocarditis or cardiomyopathy, cardiac murmurs, dysrhythmias, and signs of cardiac failure become apparent. The damage to the heart muscle can change electrical activity or lead to subacute or chronic ventricular dilation and/or systolic dysfunction.

INTERPRETATION OF LABORATORY DATA

Complete blood count may be normal, reveal neutropenia with a left shift (due to endotoxemia), or reveal neutrophilia (due to inflammation caused by bacterial infection). Cardiac failure may decrease glomerular filtration and cause hepatic congestion, thereby causing prerenal azotemia (increased SUN and creatinine) and hepatic necrosis (increased serum activity of AST and SDH). Skeletal myonecrosis resulting from toxins (monensin, lasalocid, gossypol, and *Cassia* spp.), viral infection (equine influenza), and nutritional deficiencies (vitamin E and selenium) may cause elevations in serum activity of AST and CK. Although myocardial necrosis may contribute a small amount to the elevations in these enzymes, increases in the myocardial isoenzyme CKMB are a more specific and sensitive indicator of myocardial diseases.

SIGNIFICANT DISEASES TO RULE OUT

- ◆ Electrolyte abnormalities can cause arrhythmias and systolic failure resulting from abnormalities in the serum concentrations of Na, K, Cl, tCO_2, and Ca.
- ◆ Valvular disease can lead to cardiac murmurs and failure. CKMB isoenzyme will not be increased without concurrent myocardial disease. Echocardiography may reveal the valvular abnormalities.

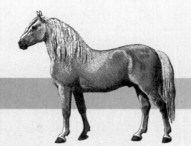

Signs

- ◆ Murmur
- ◆ Dysrhythmias
- ◆ Cardiac failure

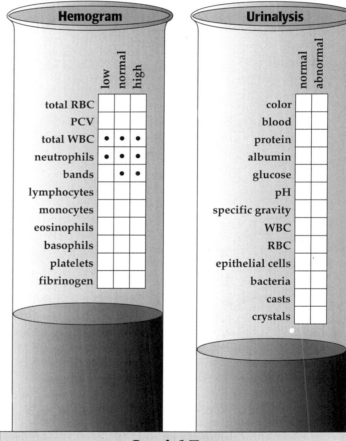

Serum Chemistry

	low	normal	high
CK		•	•
AST		•	•
SDH	•†	•†	
GGT			
bile acids			
bilirubin, total			
bilirubin, direct			
protein, total			
albumin			
globulin			
SUN	•†	•†	
creatinine	•†	•†	
glucose			
Ca			
P			
Na			
K			
Cl			
tCO$_2$			

Hemogram

	low	normal	high
total RBC			
PCV			
total WBC	•	•	•
neutrophils	•	•	•
bands		•	•
lymphocytes			
monocytes			
eosinophils			
basophils			
platelets			
fibrinogen			

Urinalysis

	normal	abnormal
color		
blood		
protein		
albumin		
glucose		
pH		
specific gravity		
WBC		
RBC		
epithelial cells		
bacteria		
casts		
crystals		

Special Tests

- ◆ Serum activity of CKMB may increase.
- ◆ Echocardiography may reveal increased cardiac dimensions and decreased fractional shortening.
- ◆ Electrocardiography may reveal arrhythmias.
- ◆ Toxicity can be evaluated by measuring amounts of ionophores in feed or intestinal contents.
- ◆ Nutritional deficiencies may result in decreased blood concentration of Se and vitamin E.

• Changes caused by the disease itself

•† Changes secondary to dysfunction caused by the disease

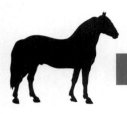

PERICARDITIS

Pericarditis, or inflammation of the pericardium, is caused by either bacterial infection (extension from pleuropneumonia or penetrating wounds) or viral infection (equine viral arteritis or equine influenza). Idiopathic pericarditis also has been described in horses. Pericarditis results in accumulation of fluid and/or exudate between the visceral and parietal pericardium. Increased pericardial pressure impairs diastolic filling of the ventricles, thereby reducing stroke volume. Cardiac failure occurs when large amounts of fluid accumulate. Clinical signs include venous distention, tachycardia, muffled heart sounds, and dependent edema.

INTERPRETATION OF LABORATORY DATA

Bacterial pericarditis occasionally causes leukocytosis, neutrophilia, and increases in plasma fibrinogen and serum globulin concentrations. Cardiac failure may decrease glomerular filtration and cause hepatic congestion, thereby causing prerenal azotemia (increased SUN and creatinine) and hepatic necrosis (increased AST and SDH). Subepicardial myocardial necrosis that sometimes accompanies pericarditis may increase the myocardial isoenzyme CKMB. Electrolyte concentrations are usually normal; however, decreased concentrations of sodium and chloride have been reported in some horses with pericarditis.

SIGNIFICANT DISEASES TO RULE OUT

◆ Myocarditis or cardiomyopathy does not muffle the heart sounds or cause echocardiographic evidence of pericardial effusion.
◆ Valvular diseases cause a murmur without muffling heart sounds. Echocardiography may reveal valvular abnormalities without evidence of pericardial effusion.

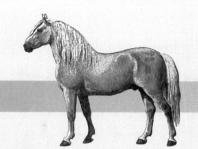

Signs

- ◆ Venous distention
- ◆ Edema
- ◆ Tachycardia
- ◆ Muffled heart sounds

Serum Chemistry

	low	normal	high
CK			
AST		•†	•†
SDH		•†	•†
GGT			
bile acids			
bilirubin, total			
bilirubin, direct			
protein, total		•	•
albumin			
globulin		•	•
SUN		•†	•†
creatinine		•†	•†
glucose			
Ca			
P			
Na	•	•	
K			
Cl	•	•	
tCO₂			

Hemogram

	low	normal	high
total RBC			
PCV			
total WBC		•	•
neutrophils		•	•
bands			
lymphocytes			
monocytes			
eosinophils			
basophils			
platelets			
fibrinogen		•	•

Urinalysis

	normal	abnormal
color		
blood		
protein		
albumin		
glucose		
pH		
specific gravity		
WBC		
RBC		
epithelial cells		
bacteria		
casts		
crystals		

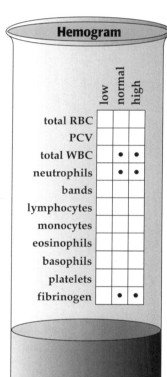
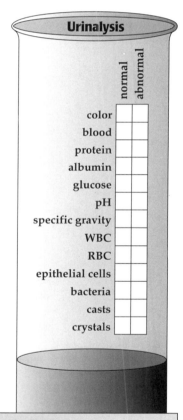

Special Tests

- ◆ Echocardiography reveals pericardial effusion.
- ◆ Microbiology sometimes reveals positive pericardial fluid cultures.
- ◆ Electrocardiogram often reveals decreased QRS amplitude and electrical alternans.
- ◆ Radiography may reveal enlarged cardiac silhouette and pleural effusion.
- ◆ Pericardial fluid cytology reveals an elevated protein concentration while the WBC count is normal or elevated.

- • Changes caused by the disease itself
- •† Changes secondary to dysfunction caused by the disease

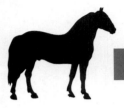

CONGENITAL CARDIOVASCULAR DISEASE

The most commonly reported congenital malformation of the heart and great vessels is ventricular septal defect (VSD). Multiple cardiac anomalies (e.g., tetralogy of Fallot), patent ductus arteriosus, truncus arteriosus (Arabian foals), tricuspid atresia, and atrial septal defects have also been reported. Animals with a small VSD may be asymptomatic. Clinical signs associated with cardiac defects include cardiac murmurs with or without a palpable thrill (holosystolic, holodiastolic, or continuous), cyanosis, exercise intolerance, and cardiac failure.

INTERPRETATION OF LABORATORY DATA

A simple VSD, patent ductus arteriosus, and atrial septal defect are not associated with any clinicopathologic abnormalities. Those anomalies associated with a right-to-left shunting of blood (tetralogy of Fallot, truncus arteriosus, and tricuspid atresia) frequently decrease arterial oxygen content. Chronic hypoxemia stimulates erythropoietin release, which promotes bone marrow erythropoiesis. Therefore, PCV, red blood cell count, and hemoglobin count are often increased (secondary polycythemia). Cardiac failure may decrease glomerular filtration and cause hepatic congestion, thereby causing prerenal azotemia (increased SUN and creatinine) and hepatic necrosis (increased AST and SDH).

SIGNIFICANT DISEASES TO RULE OUT

- ◆ Myocarditis or cardiomyopathy may also cause a cardiac murmur but is accompanied by elevation of CKMB.
- ◆ Valvular diseases (endocarditis) will increase body temperature and plasma fibrinogen concentration and result in echocardiographic evidence of vegetations.

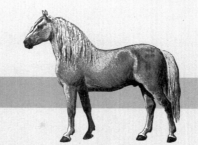

Signs

- ◆ Murmurs
- ◆ Exercise intolerance
- ◆ Cardiac failure

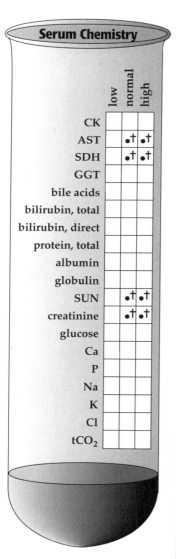

Serum Chemistry

	low	normal	high
CK			
AST	•†	•†	
SDH	•†	•†	
GGT			
bile acids			
bilirubin, total			
bilirubin, direct			
protein, total			
albumin			
globulin			
SUN	•†	•†	
creatinine	•†	•†	
glucose			
Ca			
P			
Na			
K			
Cl			
tCO₂			

Hemogram

	low	normal	high
total RBC		•	•
PCV		•	•
total WBC			
neutrophils			
bands			
lymphocytes			
monocytes			
eosinophils			
basophils			
platelets			
fibrinogen			

Urinalysis

	normal	abnormal
color		
blood		
protein		
albumin		
glucose		
pH		
specific gravity		
WBC		
RBC		
epithelial cells		
bacteria		
casts		
crystals		

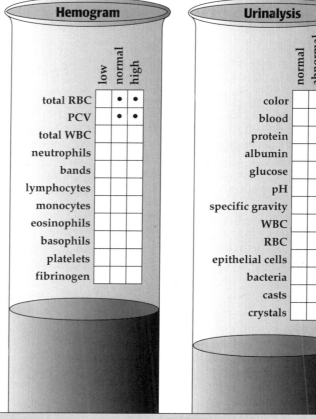

Special Tests

- ◆ Blood gas analysis sometimes reveals hypoxemia. Echocardiography reveals the cardiac anomaly or the cardiac enlargement.
- ◆ Angiocardiography and Doppler echocardiography demonstrate the abnormal flow patterns.
- ◆ Cardiac oximetry demonstrates the changes in blood oxygen tension.
- ◆ Cardiac catheterization reveals abnormal cardiac pressures.

• Changes caused by the disease itself

•† Changes secondary to dysfunction caused by the disease

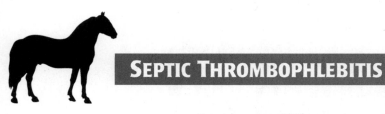

SEPTIC THROMBOPHLEBITIS

Septic venous inflammation and thrombosis due to catheterization or injection results from bacterial infection or traumatic injury of the vein. Clinical signs include swelling, vascular occlusion, fever, and pain.

INTERPRETATION OF LABORATORY DATA

Septic thrombophlebitis is accompanied by neutrophilic leukocytosis and elevation in plasma fibrinogen concentration. Nonregenerative anemia and increased serum globulin concentration occur in chronic cases.

SIGNIFICANT DISEASES TO RULE OUT

◆ Nonseptic thrombosis results in swelling and vascular occlusion without causing neutrophilic leukocytosis, increased plasma fibrinogen concentration, and fever.

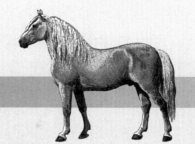

Signs

- ◆ Swelling
- ◆ Pain
- ◆ Vascular occlusion
- ◆ Fever

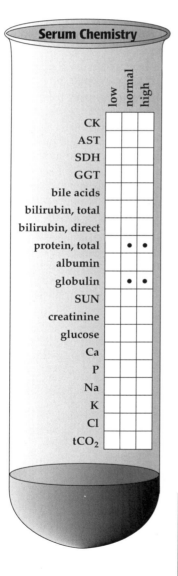

Serum Chemistry

	low	normal	high
CK			
AST			
SDH			
GGT			
bile acids			
bilirubin, total			
bilirubin, direct			
protein, total		•	•
albumin			
globulin		•	•
SUN			
creatinine			
glucose			
Ca			
P			
Na			
K			
Cl			
tCO$_2$			

Hemogram

	low	normal	high
total RBC	•	•	
PCV	•	•	
total WBC		•	•
neutrophils		•	•
bands			
lymphocytes			
monocytes			
eosinophils			
basophils			
platelets			
fibrinogen			•

Urinalysis

	normal	abnormal
color		
blood		
protein		
albumin		
glucose		
pH		
specific gravity		
WBC		
RBC		
epithelial cells		
bacteria		
casts		
crystals		

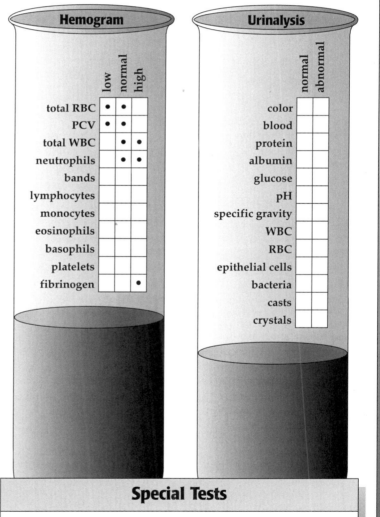

Special Tests

- ◆ Cultures of catheter tip and/or blood may reveal the bacterial etiology.
- ◆ Ultrasonography and angiography may reveal dilated vascular structures (aneurysm) or echogenic structure within blood vessel (thrombosis).

- • Changes caused by the disease itself
- •† Changes secondary to dysfunction caused by the disease

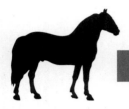

SEPTICEMIA

Bacterial infection within the bloodstream is a common cause of illness in foals. Failure of passive transfer and gastrointestinal disease are common predisposing factors. Septicemia rarely occurs in adult horses. The most common early signs of infection are lethargy, poor suckle reflex, and excessive sleeping. Fever is an uncommon clinical sign in foals with septicemia. Other signs include diarrhea, seizures, colic, uveitis, joint distention, lameness, omphalophlebitis, and respiratory distress. *Escherichia coli* is the most common causative agent.

INTERPRETATION OF LABORATORY DATA

A number of foals with septicemia have a decreased white blood cell and neutrophil count. Furthermore, most of these foals have an increased number of band neutrophils or toxic changes in the neutrophils. In foals with acute sepsis, fibrinogen concentration is commonly normal or only slightly increased. Infections of longer duration (e.g., in utero infection, osteomyelitis, arthritis, and pneumonia) frequently cause hyperfibrinogenemia, nonregenerative anemia, monocytosis, and neutrophilia. Severe cases can develop thrombocytopenia as a result of DIC. Hypoglycemia commonly accompanies neonatal sepsis, because of abnormal glucose metabolism and decreased ingestion. Decreased IgG concentrations are frequently correlated with neonatal sepsis. Hypovolemia and sepsis can result in renal and prerenal azotemia. Foals with renal azotemia have a specific gravity in the isosthenuric range (1.008 to 1.012). However, normal foals also have dilute urine. Septic shock can cause hepatocellular damage leading to increases in serum activity of AST and SDH. Renal infection can result in pyuria, hematuria, proteinuria, and the presence of urinary casts.

SIGNIFICANT DISEASES TO RULE OUT

- Neonatal isoerythrolysis causes anemia and hemoglobinuria.
- Meconium impaction can be confirmed by digital examination or abdominal radiographs.
- Prematurity can result in neutropenia and lymphopenia without increased number of band neutrophils and toxic changes.

Signs

- Lethargy
- Poor suckle reflex
- Excessive sleeping
- Fever
- Diarrhea
- Seizures
- Colic
- Uveitis
- Joint distention
- Lameness
- Respiratory distress

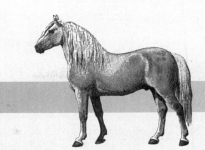

Serum Chemistry

	low	normal	high
CK			
AST		•†	•†
SDH		•†	•†
GGT			
bile acids			
bilirubin, total			
bilirubin, direct			
protein, total	•	•	
albumin			
globulin	•	•	
SUN		•	•
creatinine		•	•
glucose	•	•	
Ca			
P			
Na			
K			
Cl			
tCO₂	•	•	

Hemogram

	low	normal	high
total RBC	•	•	•
PCV	•	•	•
total WBC	•	•	•
neutrophils	•	•	•
bands		•	•
lymphocytes	•	•	
monocytes		•	•
eosinophils		•	•
basophils		•	
platelets	•	•	
fibrinogen		•	•

Urinalysis

	normal	abnormal
color		
blood	•	•
protein	•	•
albumin		
glucose		
pH		
specific gravity	•	•
WBC	•	•
RBC	•	•
epithelial cells		
bacteria		
casts	•	•
crystals		

Special Tests

- There may be radiographic evidence of pneumonia or bony infection.
- Ultrasonography may reveal omphalophlebitis.
- Positive blood cultures are obtained in the majority of cases.
- IgG concentrations are frequently decreased.

- Changes caused by the disease itself
- † Changes secondary to dysfunction caused by the disease

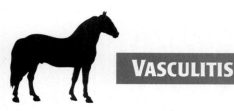

VASCULITIS

The term vasculitis refers to inflammation of blood vessels. Vasculitis may develop by direct damage from infectious agents (*Streptococcus equi*, EVA virus, EIA virus, *Ehrlichia equi*), chemicals, and endotoxins; however, it is more commonly produced via immune complex formation and deposition in the vessel wall. These complexes then activate inflammatory cells and mediators. Horses may exhibit mucosal hyperemia, petechiation, dermal or subcutaneous edema with exudation and ulceration, hematuria, and colic.

INTERPRETATION OF LABORATORY DATA

Clinical laboratory data reflect the underlying disease process. Neutrophilia, mild anemia, hyperglobulinemia, and hyperfibrinogenemia may result from the chronic inflammation. If glomerulonephritis is a part of the vasculitis, the urinalysis may show proteinuria and/or hematuria. Creatinine is usually normal unless dehydration leads to prerenal azotemia. Decreased total serum protein can occur from renal loss of albumin. Platelet counts may be mildly decreased.

Purpura hemorrhagica is thought to be a hypersensitivity vasculitis secondary to *Streptococcus equi* (strangles), and less frequently to other bacterial or viral antigens. The infective agent may be cultured if active abscesses are present, although active abscesses are not necessary for the presence of disease.

Equine viral arteritis is diagnosed by establishing seroconversion. Leukopenia with a lymphopenia may be present.

Hemolytic anemia and vasculitis associated with equine infectious anemia are confirmed by detection of specific antibodies using the agar gel immunodiffusion (Coggins) test.

The necrotizing vasculitis caused by the rickettsial agent *Ehrlichia equi* may be diagnosed by finding morula in the granulocytes of affected horses or by serologic tests using acute and convalescent serum samples.

SIGNIFICANT DISEASES TO RULE OUT

◆ Coagulation defects will reflect prolonged APTT and OSPT.
◆ Renal failure will result in isosthenuria.
◆ Thrombocytopenia or thrombocytopathy cause low platelet counts and/or abnormal platelet function tests (bleeding time).

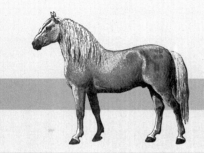

Signs

◆ Mucosal hyperemia
◆ Petechiation
◆ Dermal or subcutaneous edema with exudation and ulceration
◆ Hematuria
◆ Colic

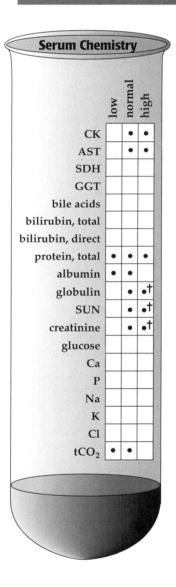

Serum Chemistry

	low	normal	high
CK		•	•
AST		•	•
SDH			
GGT			
bile acids			
bilirubin, total			
bilirubin, direct			
protein, total	•	•	•
albumin	•	•	
globulin		•	•†
SUN		•	•†
creatinine		•	•†
glucose			
Ca			
P			
Na			
K			
Cl			
tCO$_2$	•	•	

Hemogram

	low	normal	high
total RBC	•		
PCV	•		
total WBC	•	•	•
neutrophils		•	•
bands			
lymphocytes	•	•	
monocytes			
eosinophils			
basophils			
platelets	•	•	
fibrinogen			•

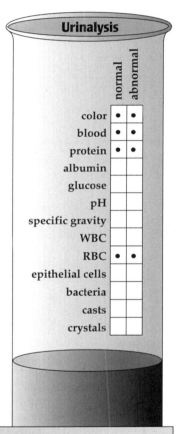

Urinalysis

	normal	abnormal
color	•	•
blood	•	•
protein	•	•
albumin		
glucose		
pH		
specific gravity		
WBC		
RBC	•	•
epithelial cells		
bacteria		
casts		
crystals		

Special Tests

◆ Coggins' test may be positive.
◆ Serum titers for rickettsial agents or EVA may be positive.
◆ ANA may reveal autoantibodies, but false positives and false negatives do occur.
◆ Culture may be positive for *Streptococcus equi*.
◆ Biopsy specimen from affected tissue will reveal vasculitis and sometimes positive immunofluorescent staining.

• Changes caused by the disease itself
•† Changes secondary to dysfunction caused by the disease

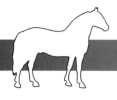

Respiratory Diseases

Pharyngitis

Guttural pouch disease

Retropharyngeal lymph node abscessation

Viral respiratory disease

Bacterial pneumonia and pleuropneumonia

Fungal pneumonia

Thoracic neoplasia

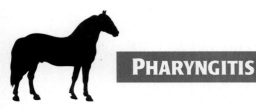

PHARYNGITIS

Pharyngitis is inflammation of the pharyngeal tissues that results from either viral infection (herpesvirus and influenza), bacterial respiratory disease (*Streptococcus* spp.), trauma (especially foreign bodies), chemical irritation, or allergy. Bilateral nasal discharge, fever, and coughing are potential signs associated with pharyngitis.

INTERPRETATION OF LABORATORY DATA

Cellulitis and abscess formation caused by foreign body penetration of the pharynx will result in hyperfibrinogenemia, nonregenerative anemia, and hyperglobulinemia. A mature neutrophilia associated with chronic inflammation is sometimes seen.

SIGNIFICANT DISEASES TO RULE OUT

- ◆ Sinusitis causes unilateral nasal discharge and radiographic evidence of fluid in the sinuses.
- ◆ Guttural pouch empyema can be diagnosed by radiography or endoscopy.

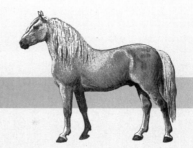

Signs

- ◆ Fever
- ◆ Coughing
- ◆ Nasal discharge

Serum Chemistry

	low	normal	high
CK			
AST			
SDH			
GGT			
bile acids			
bilirubin, total			
bilirubin, direct			
protein, total		•	•
albumin			
globulin		•	•
SUN			
creatinine			
glucose			
Ca			
P			
Na			
K			
Cl			
tCO$_2$			

Hemogram

	low	normal	high
total RBC	•	•	
PCV	•	•	
total WBC		•	•
neutrophils		•	•
bands			
lymphocytes			
monocytes			
eosinophils			
basophils			
platelets			
fibrinogen		•	•

Urinalysis

	normal	abnormal
color		
blood		
protein		
albumin		
glucose		
pH		
specific gravity		
WBC		
RBC		
epithelial cells		
bacteria		
casts		
crystals		

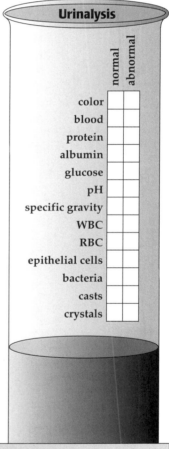

Special Tests

- ◆ Endoscopy may reveal pharyngeal lymphoid hyperplasia or pharyngeal laceration caused by foreign body.
- ◆ Radiography may allow visualization of radiodense foreign bodies.
- ◆ Culture of pharyngeal swab may allow diagnosis of *Streptococcus equi* infection.

• Changes caused by the disease itself
•† Changes secondary to dysfunction caused by the disease

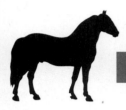

GUTTURAL POUCH DISEASE

Guttural pouch empyema is accumulation of purulent material resulting from bacterial infection. Clinical signs are unilateral or bilateral nasal discharge. Fungal infection (guttural pouch mycosis) causes epistaxis and dysphagia. *Streptococcus* spp. are common causes of empyema, and numerous fungi have been associated with mycosis, the most common being *Aspergillus nidulans*.

INTERPRETATION OF LABORATORY DATA

Inflammation caused by guttural pouch empyema or secondary aspiration pneumonia may result in leukocytosis with neutrophilia and hyperfibrinogenemia. Severe epistaxis resulting from mycosis may cause anemia and hypoproteinemia. Chronic inflammation resulting from empyema may cause hyperglobulinemia and nonregenerative anemia.

SIGNIFICANT DISEASES TO RULE OUT

◆ Retropharyngeal lymph node abscessation is diagnosed by the presence of a soft tissue mass on radiography.
◆ Bacterial pneumonia or pleuropneumonia causes the transtracheal aspirate to contain degenerative neutrophils with or without bacteria and the thoracic radiographs to demonstrate evidence of pneumonia. Thoracic auscultation may reveal abnormal lung sounds.
◆ Pharyngitis is diagnosed via endoscopy.
◆ Sinusitis is diagnosed by radiographic evidence of a fluid line in the sinuses.
◆ Ethmoidal hematoma can be diagnosed by endoscopy or radiography.

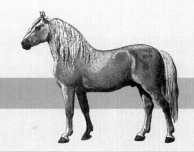

Signs

- ◆ Nasal discharge
- ◆ Epistaxis
- ◆ Dysphagia

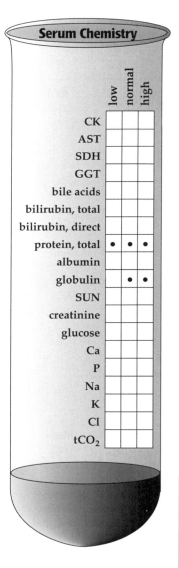

Serum Chemistry

	low	normal	high
CK			
AST			
SDH			
GGT			
bile acids			
bilirubin, total			
bilirubin, direct			
protein, total	●	●	●
albumin			
globulin		●	●
SUN			
creatinine			
glucose			
Ca			
P			
Na			
K			
Cl			
tCO₂			

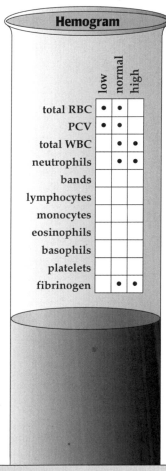

Hemogram

	low	normal	high
total RBC	●	●	
PCV	●	●	
total WBC		●	●
neutrophils		●	●
bands			
lymphocytes			
monocytes			
eosinophils			
basophils			
platelets			
fibrinogen		●	●

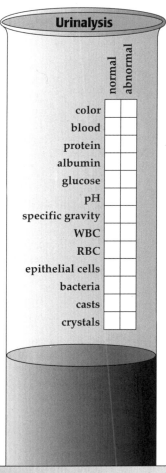

Urinalysis

	normal	abnormal
color		
blood		
protein		
albumin		
glucose		
pH		
specific gravity		
WBC		
RBC		
epithelial cells		
bacteria		
casts		
crystals		

Special Tests

- ◆ Radiography will allow identification of fluid or radiodense masses (chondroids).
- ◆ Endoscopy will allow visualization of fluid, masses, or mycosis.
- ◆ Culture of guttural pouch may identify a bacterial or fungal etiology.

● Changes caused by the disease itself

●† Changes secondary to dysfunction caused by the disease

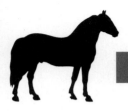

RETROPHARYNGEAL LYMPH NODE ABSCESSATION

Abscessation of the retropharyngeal lymph nodes results from *Streptococcus equi* infection, pharyngeal trauma, viral respiratory infection, or extension of guttural pouch empyema. Submandibular and sometimes retropharyngeal swelling are the clinical signs. Respiratory distress and dysphagia may result from compression of the pharynx, larynx, or nerves. Fever and depression also may occur.

INTERPRETATION OF LABORATORY DATA

Chronic inflammation associated with abscess formation may result in hyperfibrinogenemia, depression anemia, and hyperglobulinemia. Decreased feed and water intake associated with dysphagia may result in hypokalemia, hemoconcentration, and prerenal azotemia.

SIGNIFICANT DISEASES TO RULE OUT

- ◆ Lymphosarcoma is diagnosed by histopathology of biopsy sample.
- ◆ Guttural pouch empyema is diagnosed by radiography and endoscopy.

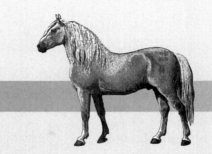

Signs

- ◆ Submandibular and retropharyngeal swelling
- ◆ Dyspnea
- ◆ Dysphagia
- ◆ Fever
- ◆ Depression

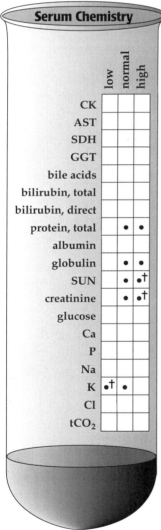

Serum Chemistry

	low	normal	high
CK			
AST			
SDH			
GGT			
bile acids			
bilirubin, total			
bilirubin, direct			
protein, total		•	•
albumin			
globulin		•	•
SUN		•	•†
creatinine		•	•†
glucose			
Ca			
P			
Na			
K	•†	•	
Cl			
tCO₂			

Hemogram

	low	normal	high
total RBC	•	•	•†
PCV	•	•	•†
total WBC		•	•
neutrophils		•	•
bands			
lymphocytes			
monocytes			
eosinophils			
basophils			
platelets			
fibrinogen		•	

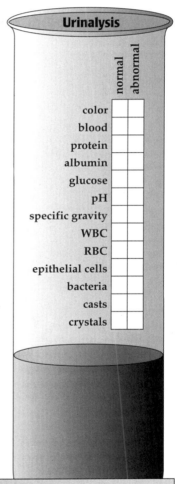

Urinalysis

	normal	abnormal
color		
blood		
protein		
albumin		
glucose		
pH		
specific gravity		
WBC		
RBC		
epithelial cells		
bacteria		
casts		
crystals		

Special Tests

- ◆ Radiography often reveals soft tissue masses.
- ◆ Endoscopy may reveal displacement of the pharynx.
- ◆ Cytology and culture of submandibular abscess reveals neutrophilic inflammation and the causative organism.

- • Changes caused by the disease itself
- •† Changes secondary to dysfunction caused by the disease

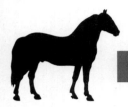

VIRAL RESPIRATORY DISEASE

Equine influenza virus and herpesvirus are the most common causes of viral respiratory disease. Although viral diseases cause lesions in the lower respiratory tract, these diseases usually present with signs attributable to upper respiratory infection. Clinical signs include fever, anorexia, depression, purulent nasal discharge, and coughing.

INTERPRETATION OF LABORATORY DATA

Early in the disease process, WBC may decrease as a result of reduced numbers of circulating lymphocytes. Influenza virus may cause myositis, thereby increasing serum CK and AST activities.

SIGNIFICANT DISEASES TO RULE OUT

◆ Bacterial pneumonia or pleuropneumonia causes the transtracheal aspirate to contain degenerative neutrophils with or without bacteria, the plasma fibrinogen concentration to be increased, and the thoracic radiographs to contain evidence of pneumonia. Thoracic auscultation may reveal abnormal lower airway sounds.
◆ *Streptococcus equi* infection causes lymph node abscessation and positive culture from a pharyngeal swab.

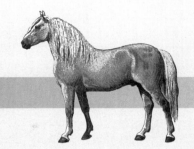

Signs

- ◆ Fever
- ◆ Depression
- ◆ Nasal discharge
- ◆ Coughing

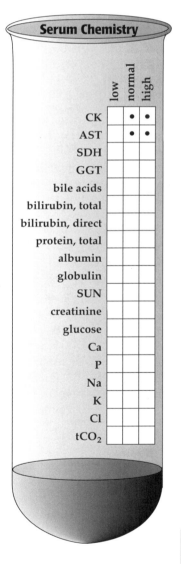

Serum Chemistry

	low	normal	high
CK		•	•
AST		•	•
SDH			
GGT			
bile acids			
bilirubin, total			
bilirubin, direct			
protein, total			
albumin			
globulin			
SUN			
creatinine			
glucose			
Ca			
P			
Na			
K			
Cl			
tCO₂			

Hemogram

	low	normal	high
total RBC			
PCV			
total WBC		•	•
neutrophils			
bands			
lymphocytes		•	•
monocytes			
eosinophils			
basophils			
platelets			
fibrinogen			

Urinalysis

	normal	abnormal
color		
blood		
protein		
albumin		
glucose		
pH		
specific gravity		
WBC		
RBC		
epithelial cells		
bacteria		
casts		
crystals		

Special Tests

- ◆ A fourfold rise in antibody titer over a 2-week period is suggestive of recent infection.

• Changes caused by the disease itself

•† Changes secondary to dysfunction caused by the disease

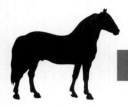

BACTERIAL PNEUMONIA AND PLEUROPNEUMONIA

Streptococcus zooepidemicus is the most common cause of septic inflammation of the lungs and pleura. *Pasteurella* sp., *Klebsiella* sp., *Escherichia coli*, *Bordetella bronchiseptica*, *Actinobacillus* sp., *Actinobacillus suis*, *Clostridium* sp., and *Bacteroides* sp are common complicating organisms. *E. coli* and *Actinobacillus equuli* may cause pneumonia in foals as a consequence of generalized septicemia. *Rhodococcus equi* is a common cause of pneumonia and pulmonary abscessation in foals two to five months of age. Increased body temperature, increased respiratory rate, coughing, and abnormal lung sounds are common clinical findings.

INTERPRETATION OF LABORATORY DATA

Decreased food and water intake caused by depression commonly result in hypokalemia and hemoconcentration (increased PCV and total serum protein concentration) and prerenal azotemia (increased SUN and creatinine). The septic inflammation associated with pneumonia and pleuropneumonia frequently increases the plasma fibrinogen concentration. Peripheral WBC and neutrophil counts are less commonly increased. Neutrophil consumption and endotoxemia sometimes decrease neutrophil count and increase band count. In chronic cases, increased serum globulin concentration and nonregenerative anemia occur.

SIGNIFICANT DISEASES TO RULE OUT

- Chronic obstructive pulmonary disease does not alter plasma fibrinogen concentration or serum globulin concentration. Transtracheal aspirate contains increased numbers of nondegenerate neutrophils and sometimes eosinophils without bacteria. Thoracic radiography and ultrasonography are normal or reveal diffuse bronchiolar infiltrates.
- Viral respiratory disease does not alter either plasma fibrinogen or serum globulin concentration. Thoracic auscultation reveals sounds consistent with upper airway disease. Thoracic radiography and ultrasonography are normal.

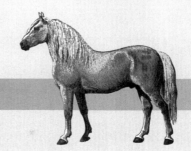

Signs

- ◆ Fever
- ◆ Tachypnea
- ◆ Coughing
- ◆ Abnormal lung sounds

Serum Chemistry

	low	normal	high
CK			
AST			
SDH			
GGT			
bile acids			
bilirubin, total			
bilirubin, direct			
protein, total		•	•
albumin			
globulin		•	•
SUN		•	•†
creatinine		•	•†
glucose			
Ca			
P			
Na			
K	•†	•	
Cl			
tCO$_2$			

Hemogram

	low	normal	high
total RBC	•	•	•†
PCV	•	•	•†
total WBC	•	•	•
neutrophils	•	•	
bands		•	•
lymphocytes			
monocytes			
eosinophils			
basophils			
platelets			
fibrinogen		•	

Urinalysis

	normal	abnormal
color		
blood		
protein		
albumin		
glucose		
pH		
specific gravity		
WBC		
RBC		
epithelial cells		
bacteria		
casts		
crystals		

Special Tests

- ◆ Transtracheal fluid and pleural fluid cytology reveals increased numbers of neutrophils, which may be degenerate, with or without bacteria.
- ◆ Microbiology frequently yields positive cultures and positive gram staining of transtracheal aspirate and pleural fluid.
- ◆ Radiography reveals interstitial or peribronchial infiltrates (especially ventral thorax).
- ◆ Ultrasonography reveals pleural fluid and pulmonary atelectasis, consolidation, or abscessation.

• Changes caused by the disease itself

•† Changes secondary to dysfunction caused by the disease

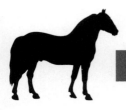

FUNGAL PNEUMONIA

Fungi are ubiquitous in the environment, but are a rare cause of pneumonia in horses. Clinical signs include increased body temperature and respiratory rate, coughing, purulent nasal exudate sometimes containing blood, and abnormal lung sounds. Fungal pneumonia usually occurs secondary to other debilitating illness (e.g., acute enterocolitis) or severe stress. Opportunistic fungi such as *Aspergillus* spp., *Mucor* spp., and *Candida* spp. usually infect only immunocompromised patients. Pathogenic fungi such as *Coccidioides immitis*, *Histoplasma capsulatum*, and *Cryptococcus neoformans* may infect horses that are immunocompetent.

INTERPRETATION OF LABORATORY DATA

In acute fulminant cases, WBC demonstrates leukopenia, neutropenia, and a left shift. The inflammatory disease increases plasma fibrinogen concentration. Leukocytosis resulting from neutrophilia, increased serum globulin and total protein concentration, and nonregenerative anemia may occur in chronic cases.

SIGNIFICANT DISEASES TO RULE OUT

◆ Bacterial pneumonia causes the transtracheal aspirate to contain neutrophilic inflammation without fungal hyphae.

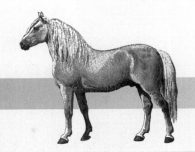

Signs

- ◆ Fever
- ◆ Tachypnea
- ◆ Coughing
- ◆ Abnormal lung sounds

Serum Chemistry

	low	normal	high
CK			
AST			
SDH			
GGT			
bile acids			
bilirubin, total			
bilirubin, direct			
protein, total		•	•
albumin			
globulin		•	•
SUN			
creatinine			
glucose			
Ca			
P			
Na			
K			
Cl			
tCO$_2$			

Hemogram

	low	normal	high
total RBC	•	•	
PCV	•	•	
total WBC	•	•	•
neutrophils	•	•	•
bands		•	•
lymphocytes			
monocytes			
eosinophils			
basophils			
platelets			
fibrinogen		•	•

Urinalysis

	normal	abnormal
color		
blood		
protein		
albumin		
glucose		
pH		
specific gravity		
WBC		
RBC		
epithelial cells		
bacteria		
casts		
crystals		

Special Tests

- ◆ Radiography reveals patchy bronchopneumonia.
- ◆ Cytology of transtracheal aspirate or histopathology of biopsy reveals large numbers of fungal hyphae in association with neutrophilic and mononuclear inflammation.
- ◆ Microbiology reveals culture of fungal organisms from transtracheal aspirate (opportunistic fungi can be cultured from transtracheal aspirate of normal horses).

● Changes caused by the disease itself
●† Changes secondary to dysfunction caused by the disease

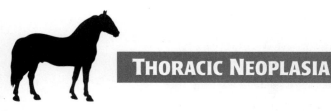

THORACIC NEOPLASIA

Although the incidence of thoracic neoplasia in horses is low, numerous tumor types have been reported, including primary thoracic tumors (lymphosarcoma, pleural mesothelioma, chondrosarcoma, and thymoma), primary pulmonary tumors (granular cell tumor, bronchial myxoma, and pulmonary carcinoma), and metastatic tumors (squamous cell carcinoma, hemangiosarcoma, and metastatic adenocarcinoma). Lymphosarcoma is the single most common neoplasia of the thorax. Clinical signs include weight loss, anorexia, tachypnea, abnormal lung sounds resulting from pleural effusion, dependent edema, and jugular distention.

INTERPRETATION OF LABORATORY DATA

Increased serum globulins and nonregenerative anemia may occur in chronic cases. Inflammation resulting from tumor necrosis can lead to neutrophilia and leukocytosis. Plasma fibrinogen may be increased, but is frequently normal. Hypoalbuminemia may result from loss in pleural effusion.

SIGNIFICANT DISEASES TO RULE OUT

◆ Bacterial pneumonia or pleuropneumonia is not accompanied by neoplastic cells on cytology or histopathology.

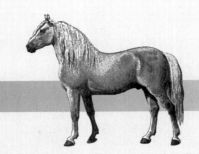

Signs

◆ Weight loss
◆ Anorexia
◆ Tachypnea
◆ Abnormal lung sounds
◆ Dependent edema
◆ Jugular pulsation

Serum Chemistry

	low	normal	high
CK			
AST			
SDH			
GGT			
bile acids			
bilirubin, total			
bilirubin, direct			
protein, total		•	•
albumin	•	•	
globulin		•	•
SUN			
creatinine			
glucose			
Ca			
P			
Na			
K			
Cl			
tCO$_2$			

Hemogram

	low	normal	high
total RBC	•	•	
PCV	•	•	
total WBC		•	•
neutrophils		•	•
bands			
lymphocytes			
monocytes			
eosinophils			
basophils			
platelets			
fibrinogen		•	•

Urinalysis

	normal	abnormal
color		
blood		
protein		
albumin		
glucose		
pH		
specific gravity		
WBC		
RBC		
epithelial cells		
bacteria		
casts		
crystals		

Special Tests

◆ Cytology of pleural fluid, needle aspirates of superficial pulmonary masses, or tracheobronchial aspirates may reveal neoplastic cells.
◆ Radiography may reveal nodular masses.
◆ Ultrasonography may identify pulmonary masses that extend to the pleural surface.
◆ Histopathology of accessible thoracic masses or involved peripheral lymph nodes (lymphosarcoma) may be diagnostic.

• Changes caused by the disease itself
•† Changes secondary to dysfunction caused by the disease

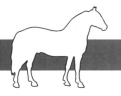

Gastrointestinal Diseases

Gastroduodenal ulceration

Gastric neoplasia

Duodenitis/proximal jejunitis

Nonstrangulating obstruction of the small intestine

Strangulating obstruction of the small intestine

Nonstrangulating obstruction of the large intestine

Strangulating obstruction of the large intestine

Nonstrangulating infarction

Peritonitis

Acute colitis

Foal diarrhea

Cantharidin toxicity (blister beetle)

Nonsteroidal antiinflammatory drug (NSAID) toxicity

Intestinal neoplasia

Parasitism

Intraabdominal abscessation

Granulomatous, eosinophilic, lymphocytic, and basophilic
enteritis

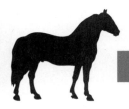

GASTRODUODENAL ULCERATION

Gastroduodenal ulceration is an inflammatory lesion of the mucous membrane for which the specific etiology is unknown. Gastric acid hypersecretion, disturbances of mucosal blood flow, and motility disorders are potentially involved in the initiation and perpetuation of ulceration. Other disease processes (foal diarrhea and neonatal sepsis) and stressful conditions (horses in active training) are factors commonly associated with a higher incidence of ulceration. Many animals with ulceration are asymptomatic. In symptomatic animals, signs include diarrhea, poor growth, abdominal pain, salivation, and bruxism. Duodenal ulceration can lead to cholangitis resulting from retrograde infection of the bile duct. Ulceration occasionally progresses to pyloric or duodenal stenosis.

INTERPRETATION OF LABORATORY DATA

Hematologic counts are usually normal. Lesions can occasionally result in hemorrhage that usually is not associated with anemia or hypoproteinemia. In foals, anorexia caused by abdominal pain may result in hypoglycemia, hypokalemia, and prerenal azotemia (increased SUN and creatinine). Concurrent disease processes may decrease serum electrolyte concentration (diarrhea) and neutrophil count (sepsis). Cholangitis causes elevation of serum GGT activity.

SIGNIFICANT DISEASES TO RULE OUT

◆ Salmonellosis is diagnosed by culture of *Salmonella* organisms from feces. Gastric ulceration can accompany *Salmonella*-induced diarrhea and can be diagnosed by endoscopy or response to antiulcer medication.
◆ Rotavirus is confirmed by identification of virus in feces via ELISA (Rotazyme, Abbott Laboratories), latex agglutination (Virogen Rotatest, Wampole Laboratories), or electron microscopy. Gastric ulceration can accompany *Salmonella*-induced diarrhea and can be diagnosed by endoscopy or response to antiulcer medication.
◆ Small intestine obstruction will result in small intestinal distention, identified by radiography or rectal examination.

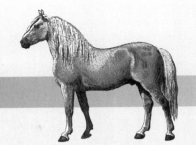

Signs

- ◆ Diarrhea
- ◆ Poor growth
- ◆ Abdominal pain
- ◆ Salivation
- ◆ Bruxism

Serum Chemistry

	low	normal	high
CK			
AST			
SDH			
GGT		•	•
bile acids			
bilirubin, total			
bilirubin, direct			
protein, total			
albumin			
globulin			
SUN		•	•†
creatinine		•	•†
glucose	•†	•	
Ca			
P			
Na	•	•	
K	•	•	
Cl	•	•	
tCO$_2$	•	•	

Hemogram

	low	normal	high
total RBC			
PCV			
total WBC	•	•	
neutrophils	•	•	
bands		•	•
lymphocytes			
monocytes			
eosinophils			
basophils			
platelets			
fibrinogen			

Urinalysis

	normal	abnormal
color		
blood		
protein		
albumin		
glucose		
pH		
specific gravity		
WBC		
RBC		
epithelial cells		
bacteria		
casts		
crystals		

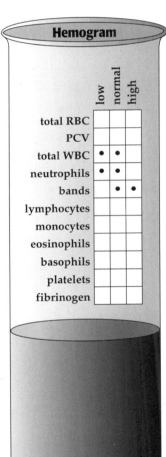
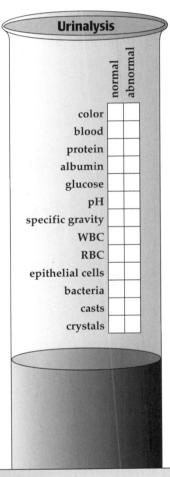

Special Tests

- ◆ Gastroscopy will reveal the ulceration of the squamous or glandular mucosa.
- ◆ Radiography (foals) of the abdomen may reveal gastric distention.
- ◆ Contrast radiography (foals) may reveal pyloric stenosis.

• Changes caused by the disease itself
•† Changes secondary to dysfunction caused by the disease

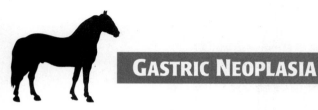

GASTRIC NEOPLASIA

Neoplastic diseases of the equine stomach include squamous cell carcinoma, lymphosarcoma, mesothelioma, and gastric adenocarcinoma. Squamous-cell carcinoma is by far the most common gastric neoplasm. Squamous-cell carcinoma occurs in older horses and originates in the gastric squamous epithelium. These tumors either metastasize, cause gastrointestinal bleeding, or obstruct the cardia. Thoracic metastasis often causes pleural effusion. Presenting signs include weight loss, dyspnea, anemia, nasal reflux, and colic.

INTERPRETATION OF LABORATORY DATA

Nonregenerative anemia resulting from chronic disease is common in horses with gastric neoplasia. Rarely, blood loss caused by ulceration and bleeding into the stomach may result in anemia and hypoproteinemia. Hypokalemia is common, because of decreased food intake. Severe inflammation associated with metastasis may increase plasma fibrinogen.

SIGNIFICANT DISEASES TO RULE OUT

- Gastric ulceration is differentiated by visualization on gastroscopy and response to medication.
- Intestinal parasitism will improve after larvacidal anthelmintic therapy.

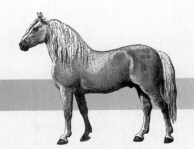

Signs

- ◆ Weight loss
- ◆ Anemia
- ◆ Nasal reflux
- ◆ Colic

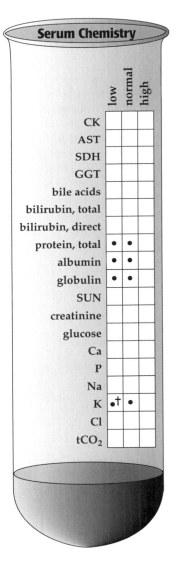

Serum Chemistry

	low	normal	high
CK			
AST			
SDH			
GGT			
bile acids			
bilirubin, total			
bilirubin, direct			
protein, total	●	●	
albumin	●	●	
globulin	●	●	
SUN			
creatinine			
glucose			
Ca			
P			
Na			
K	●†	●	
Cl			
tCO₂			

Hemogram

	low	normal	high
total RBC	●		
PCV	●		
total WBC			
neutrophils			
bands			
lymphocytes			
monocytes			
eosinophils			
basophils			
platelets			
fibrinogen		●	●

Urinalysis

	normal	abnormal
color		
blood		
protein		
albumin		
glucose		
pH		
specific gravity		
WBC		
RBC		
epithelial cells		
bacteria		
casts		
crystals		

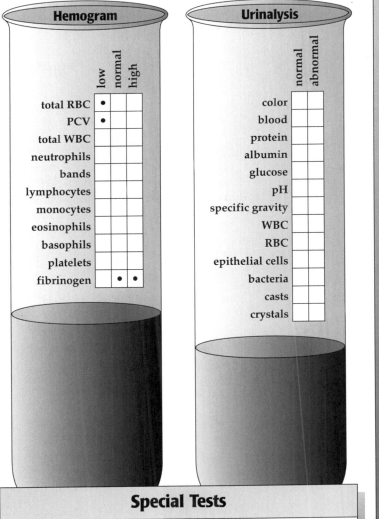

Special Tests

- ◆ Abdominal or thoracic fluid cytology may reveal neoplastic squamous cells.
- ◆ Gastroscopy allows visualization and biopsy of the mass.

● Changes caused by the disease itself
●† Changes secondary to dysfunction caused by the disease

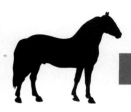

DUODENITIS/PROXIMAL JEJUNITIS

This is a syndrome characterized by transmural inflammation, edema, and hemorrhage in the duodenum and proximal jejunum. *Clostridium* and *Salmonella* are sometimes incriminated. The cause of the extensive intestinal inflammation is unknown. Clinically relevant events that result from the intestinal damage are abdominal pain, small intestinal distention, profuse nasogastric reflux, hypovolemia, and endotoxic shock. The abdominal pain typically resolves after gastric decompression via a nasogastric tube and is replaced by signs of depression.

INTERPRETATION OF LABORATORY DATA

Typical clinical laboratory findings include an increased packed cell volume and serum protein resulting from hemoconcentration, increased creatinine and SUN concentration resulting from prerenal or renal azotemia, and hypokalemia resulting from decreased feed intake. Hyponatremia, hypochloridemia, and alkalosis may develop. Poor perfusion resulting from hypovolemia and endotoxic shock also causes metabolic acidosis (decreased total CO_2). CBC may reveal a normal, increased (neutrophilia due to inflammation), or decreased (neutropenia and left shift due to endotoxemia and sequestration) WBC. Renal azotemia is accompanied by isosthenuric specific gravity (1.008 to 1.012) and sometimes blood, protein, and casts in the urine.

SIGNIFICANT DISEASES TO RULE OUT

◆ Nonstrangulating obstruction differs in that the signs of abdominal pain are more persistent. Abdominal fluid and complete blood count are usually normal.

◆ Strangulating obstruction results in a rapid onset of shock, persistent abdominal pain, and severe distention of small intestine on rectal examination. Abdominal fluid may be sanguineous or have an increased cell count and protein content.

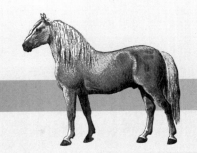

Signs

- ◆ Abdominal pain
- ◆ Depression
- ◆ Small intestinal distention
- ◆ Nasogastric reflux
- ◆ Hypovolemia
- ◆ Endotoxic shock

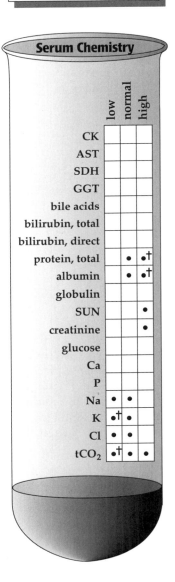

Serum Chemistry

	low	normal	high
CK			
AST			
SDH			
GGT			
bile acids			
bilirubin, total			
bilirubin, direct			
protein, total		•	•†
albumin		•	•†
globulin			
SUN			•
creatinine			•
glucose			
Ca			
P			
Na	•	•	
K	•†	•	
Cl	•	•	
tCO$_2$	•†	•	•

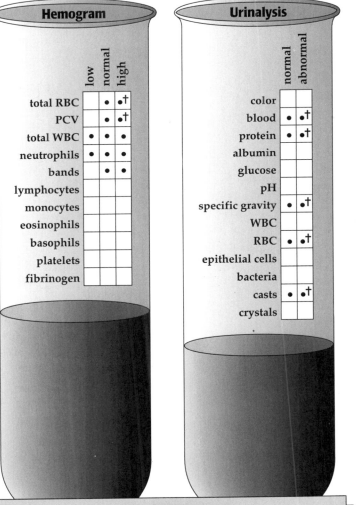

Hemogram

	low	normal	high
total RBC		•	•†
PCV		•	•†
total WBC	•	•	•
neutrophils	•	•	•
bands		•	•
lymphocytes			
monocytes			
eosinophils			
basophils			
platelets			
fibrinogen			

Urinalysis

	normal	abnormal
color		
blood	•	•†
protein	•	•†
albumin		
glucose		
pH		
specific gravity	•	•†
WBC		
RBC	•	•†
epithelial cells		
bacteria		
casts	•	•†
crystals		

Special Tests

- ◆ Abdominal fluid cytology reveals elevated protein concentration and sometimes increased WBC.
- ◆ Fecal culture sometimes reveals *Salmonella*.

- • Changes caused by the disease itself
- •† Changes secondary to dysfunction caused by the disease

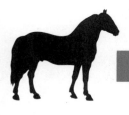

NONSTRANGULATING OBSTRUCTION
OF THE SMALL INTESTINE

Ascarid impaction, ileal impaction, ileal hypertrophy, and intraabdominal adhesions are potential causes of small intestinal obstruction that does not obstruct blood flow. Nonstrangulating obstruction may result in partial obstruction but usually causes complete luminal obstruction. Complete obstruction causes acute abdominal pain, often with nasogastric reflux. Transrectal examination reveals distended small intestine. Partial obstruction of the small intestine may cause chronic weight loss, lethargy, and intermittent signs of mild to moderate abdominal pain.

INTERPRETATION OF LABORATORY DATA

Serum chemistry and hematology are often normal. Hypovolemia may result in hemoconcentration (increased packed cell volume and serum protein concentration) and prerenal or renal azotemia (increased SUN and creatinine concentration). Renal azotemia is accompanied by isosthenuric specific gravity (1.008 to 1.012) and sometimes blood, protein, and casts in the urine. Decreased feed intake results in hypokalemia. Long-standing obstruction may lead to mucosal damage. The end result of mucosal damage can be neutropenia, left shift, and toxic changes caused by endotoxemia and hypoproteinemia caused by mucosal exudation of protein.

SIGNIFICANT DISEASES TO RULE OUT

- Duodenitis/proximal jejunitis causes profuse nasogastric reflux and abdominal pain that usually resolves after nasogastric decompression and is replaced by depression. Abdominal fluid protein concentration and nucleated cell count are often increased.
- Strangulating obstruction causes severe persistent abdominal pain, rapid progression of shock, and severe distention of small intestine on rectal examination. Abdominal fluid is sometimes serosanguineous, with increased protein concentration and cell count.

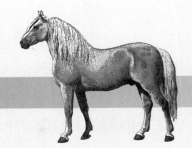

Signs

◆ Abdominal pain
◆ Nasogastric reflux
◆ Small intestinal distention

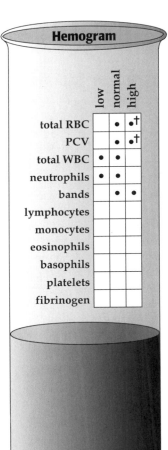

Serum Chemistry

	low	normal	high
CK			
AST			
SDH			
GGT			
bile acids			
bilirubin, total			
bilirubin, direct			
protein, total	•	•	•†
albumin	•	•	•†
globulin	•	•	•†
SUN		•	•†
creatinine		•	•†
glucose			
Ca			
P			
Na			
K	•†	•	
Cl			
tCO₂			

Hemogram

	low	normal	high
total RBC		•	•†
PCV		•	•†
total WBC	•	•	
neutrophils	•	•	
bands		•	•
lymphocytes			
monocytes			
eosinophils			
basophils			
platelets			
fibrinogen			

Urinalysis

	normal	abnormal
color		
blood		•†
protein	•	•†
albumin		
glucose		
pH		
specific gravity	•	•†
WBC		
RBC	•	•†
epithelial cells		
bacteria		
casts	•	•†
crystals		

Special Tests

◆ Abdominal fluid cytology is usually normal except in long-standing cases that lead to compromise of the bowel wall.
◆ Abdominal radiography (foals) reveals moderate small intestinal distention.

• Changes caused by the disease itself
•† Changes secondary to dysfunction caused by the disease

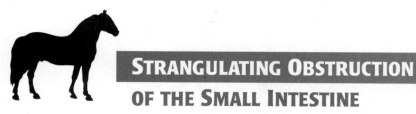

STRANGULATING OBSTRUCTION
OF THE SMALL INTESTINE

Strangulating obstruction causes complete intestinal luminal obstruction combined with significant vascular compromise. The hypoxia and ischemia that develop lead to necrosis of the involved segment of intestine. As a result of ischemia, severe unrelenting abdominal pain and hypovolemic and endotoxic shock develop rapidly. Causes include volvulus, lipomas, intussusception, and herniation.

INTERPRETATION OF LABORATORY DATA

Loss of fluid from the vascular space results in hemoconcentration (increased PCV and serum protein concentration) and hypovolemic shock. In long-standing cases, loss of protein into the peritoneal cavity and interstitial space results in a decreased serum protein concentration. Poor perfusion resulting from hypovolemia and endotoxic shock causes prerenal or renal azotemia (increased SUN and creatinine concentration) and metabolic acidosis (decreased total CO_2). Stress and endotoxemia may increase the blood glucose concentration; however, the blood glucose concentration decreases during some stages of endotoxemia. CBC sometimes reveals increased WBC as a result of a neutrophilia caused by stress. However, endotoxemia (especially after surgical correction of strangulation) can lead to leukopenia, neutropenia (due to margination of neutrophils), and left shift. Renal azotemia is accompanied by isosthenuric specific gravity (1.008 to 1.012) and sometimes blood, protein, and casts in the urine. Poor perfusion may lead to centrilobular necrosis and increased SDH and AST.

SIGNIFICANT DISEASES TO RULE OUT

- Duodenitis/proximal jejunitis causes profuse nasogastric reflux and abdominal pain that is replaced with depression after nasogastric decompression.
- Nonstrangulating obstruction causes a slower progression of shock, intestinal distention, and pain. Abdominal fluid is usually normal.

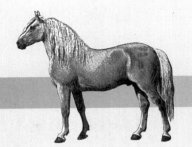

Signs

- ◆ Abdominal pain
- ◆ Hypovolemic and endotoxic shock

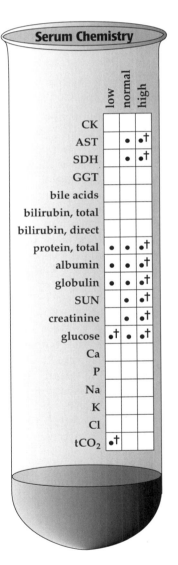

Serum Chemistry

	low	normal	high
CK			•
AST		•	•†
SDH		•	•†
GGT			
bile acids			
bilirubin, total			
bilirubin, direct			
protein, total	•	•	•†
albumin	•	•	•†
globulin	•	•	•†
SUN		•	•†
creatinine		•	•†
glucose	•†	•	•†
Ca			
P			
Na			
K			
Cl			
tCO$_2$	•†		

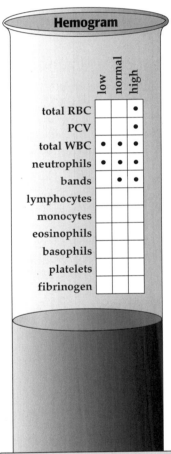

Hemogram

	low	normal	high
total RBC			•
PCV			•
total WBC	•	•	•
neutrophils	•	•	•
bands		•	•
lymphocytes			
monocytes			
eosinophils			
basophils			
platelets			
fibrinogen			

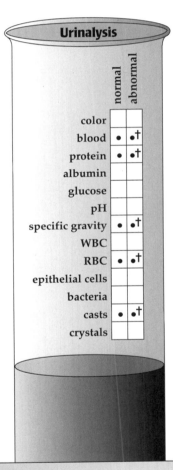

Urinalysis

	normal	abnormal
color		
blood	•	•†
protein	•	•†
albumin		
glucose		
pH		
specific gravity	•	•†
WBC		
RBC	•	•†
epithelial cells		
bacteria		
casts	•	•†
crystals		

Special Tests

- ◆ Cytology of abdominal fluid may reveal sanguineous fluid with increased protein concentration and variably increased neutrophil count.
- ◆ Ultrasonography of the abdomen in foals may reveal an intussusception.
- ◆ Radiography of the abdomen in foals will reveal moderate to severe small intestinal distention.

- • Changes caused by the disease itself
- •† Changes secondary to dysfunction caused by the disease

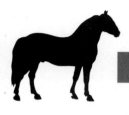

NONSTRANGULATING OBSTRUCTION
OF THE LARGE INTESTINE

Cecum or colon impaction, enteroliths, neoplasia, adhesions, and displacements are potential causes of large intestinal obstruction that does not impair blood flow. Anorexia, abdominal distention, decreased fecal passage, colon distention, and mild to severe abdominal pain result. Rectal examination reveals large intestinal distention and sometimes the cause of the obstruction (e.g., impaction, displacement, or adhesions).

INTERPRETATION OF LABORATORY DATA

Packed cell volume and serum protein concentration may be increased as a result of hemoconcentration. Creatinine and SUN may be increased because of hypovolemia, thereby causing prerenal or renal azotemia. Concurrent infection with *Salmonella* spp. may cause neutropenia and a left shift. In addition, neutrophil count may be decreased in long-standing cases, because of damage to the intestinal mucosa, thereby allowing absorption of endotoxin. Mucosal exudation of protein in these long-standing cases may lead to hypoproteinemia. Metabolic alkalosis (increased total CO_2) sometimes accompanies nonstrangulating large colon obstruction. Biliary obstruction may lead to increases in the serum activity of GGT. Renal azotemia is accompanied by isosthenuric specific gravity (1.008 to 1.012) and sometimes blood, protein, and casts in the urine. Decreased food intake leads to hypokalemia.

SIGNIFICANT DISEASES TO RULE OUT

◆ Strangulating obstruction causes unrelenting abdominal pain and more severe distention of large intestine on rectal examination. Abdominal fluid is sometimes serosanguineous, with increased protein concentration and cell count.

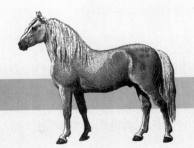

Signs

- Anorexia
- Decreased fecal passage
- Colon distention
- Abdominal pain

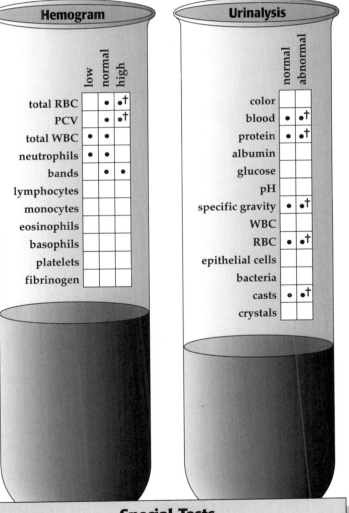

Serum Chemistry

	low	normal	high
CK			
AST			
SDH			
GGT		•	•
bile acids			
bilirubin, total			
bilirubin, direct			
protein, total	•	•	•†
albumin	•	•	•†
globulin	•	•	•†
SUN		•	•†
creatinine		•	•†
glucose			
Ca			
P			
Na			
K	•†	•	
Cl			
tCO$_2$		•	•

Hemogram

	low	normal	high
total RBC		•	•†
PCV		•	•†
total WBC	•	•	
neutrophils	•	•	
bands		•	•
lymphocytes			
monocytes			
eosinophils			
basophils			
platelets			
fibrinogen			

Urinalysis

	normal	abnormal
color		
blood	•	•†
protein	•	•†
albumin		
glucose		
pH		
specific gravity	•	•†
WBC		
RBC	•	•†
epithelial cells		
bacteria		
casts	•	•†
crystals		

Special Tests

- Abdominal fluid cytology remains normal except in long-standing cases that lead to compromise of the bowel wall.

• Changes caused by the disease itself
•† Changes secondary to dysfunction caused by the disease

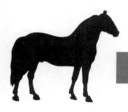

STRANGULATING OBSTRUCTION
OF THE LARGE INTESTINE

Strangulating obstructions cause complete luminal obstruction combined with significant compromise of the vascular integrity of the intestine. Severe unrelenting abdominal pain and hypovolemic and endotoxic shock develop rapidly in horses with strangulating obstructions. Large intestinal strangulating obstructions include large intestinal torsion, intussusception, and incarceration through mesenteric defects. The hypoxia and ischemia that develop lead to necrosis of the involved segment of intestine.

INTERPRETATION OF LABORATORY DATA

The ensuing shock causes a rapidly progressive hemoconcentration (increased PCV and serum protein concentration). In long-standing cases, loss of protein into the interstitial spaces and peritoneal cavity decreases serum protein concentration. However, in the face of hemoconcentration, serum protein concentration may be normal. Metabolic acidosis (decreased serum total CO_2) may occur in horses with poor perfusion resulting from shock. Stress and endotoxemia may increase the blood glucose concentration; however, the blood glucose concentration decreases during some stages of endotoxemia. CBC sometimes reveals increased WBC as a result of neutrophilia caused by stress. Endotoxemia (especially after surgical correction of strangulation) can lead to neutropenia (due to margination of neutrophils) and left shift. Poor perfusion may lead to centrilobular necrosis, which increases serum SDH and AST activity. Large colon obstruction may lead to biliary obstruction, which increases serum GGT activity. Hypovolemia and shock can result in prerenal or renal azotemia. Renal azotemia is accompanied by isosthenuric specific gravity (1.008 to 1.012) and sometimes blood, protein, and casts in the urine.

SIGNIFICANT DISEASES TO RULE OUT

◆ Nonstrangulating obstruction causes slow progression of shock, intestinal distention, and pain. Abdominal fluid is usually normal.

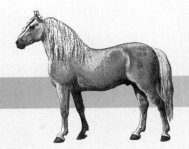

Signs

- ◆ Abdominal pain
- ◆ Hypovolemic and endotoxic shock
- ◆ Colon distention

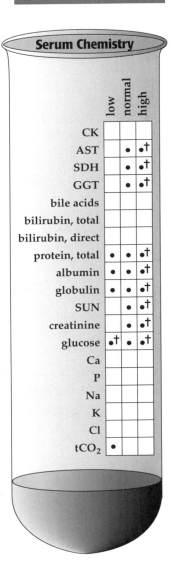

Serum Chemistry

	low	normal	high
CK			
AST		•	•†
SDH		•	•†
GGT		•	•†
bile acids			
bilirubin, total			
bilirubin, direct			
protein, total	•	•	•†
albumin	•	•	•†
globulin	•	•	•†
SUN		•	•†
creatinine		•	•†
glucose	•†	•	•†
Ca			
P			
Na			
K			
Cl			
tCO₂	•		

Hemogram

	low	normal	high
total RBC		•	•†
PCV		•	•†
total WBC	•	•	•
neutrophils	•	•	•
bands		•	•
lymphocytes			
monocytes			
eosinophils			
basophils			
platelets			
fibrinogen			

Urinalysis

	normal	abnormal
color		
blood	•	•†
protein	•	•†
albumin		
glucose		
pH		
specific gravity	•	•†
WBC		
RBC	•	•†
epithelial cells		
bacteria		
casts	•	•†
crystals		

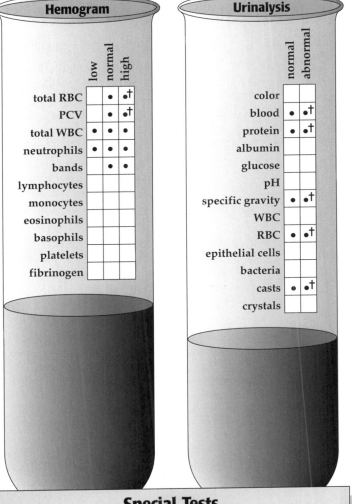

Special Tests

- ◆ Abdominal fluid may be sanguineous with increased protein concentration; increased neutrophil count in abdominal fluid is variable.

- • Changes caused by the disease itself
- •† Changes secondary to dysfunction caused by the disease

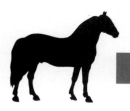

Nonstrangulating Infarction

This term describes infarction (necrosis resulting from loss of blood supply) of the intestine without a constricting or compressive lesion. Potential clinical findings are abdominal pain, hypovolemic and endotoxic shock, fever, diarrhea, and nasogastric reflux. Infarction is most likely the result of hypoxia induced by vasospasm. Infestation with the fourth and fifth stages of *Strongylus vulgaris* larvae may be involved in the pathogenesis of nonstrangulating infarction.

Interpretation of Laboratory Data

Loss of fluid into the intestinal lumen and decreased fluid intake lead to hemoconcentration (increased PCV and serum protein concentration), thereby causing prerenal or renal (increased creatinine and SUN concentration) azotemia. Renal azotemia is accompanied by isosthenuric specific gravity (1.008 to 1.012) and sometimes blood, protein, and casts in the urine. Serum protein concentration may be increased as a result of chronic inflammation caused by parasitism or decreased as a result of protein loss through damaged intestinal mucosa. The complete blood count may reveal either decreased (neutropenia with a left shift due to endotoxemia), normal, or increased (neutrophilia due to inflammation) WBC.

Significant Diseases to Rule Out

◆ Nonstrangulating obstruction does not usually cause changes in the abdominal fluid.
◆ Strangulating obstruction causes severe distention of large intestine on rectal exam.
◆ Colitis often results in decreased serum concentrations of sodium, chloride, potassium, and total CO_2. Abdominal fluid WBC and protein concentration are normal.

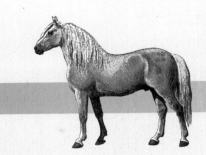

Signs

- Abdominal pain
- Hypovolemic and endotoxic shock
- Fever
- Diarrhea
- Nasogastric reflux

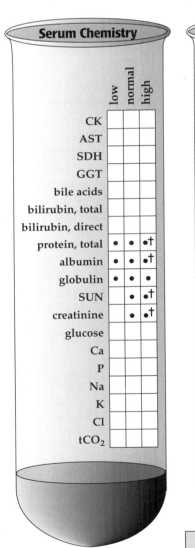

Serum Chemistry

	low	normal	high
CK			
AST			
SDH			
GGT			
bile acids			
bilirubin, total			
bilirubin, direct			
protein, total	•	•	•†
albumin	•	•	•†
globulin	•	•	•
SUN		•	•†
creatinine		•	•†
glucose			
Ca			
P			
Na			
K			
Cl			
tCO₂			

Hemogram

	low	normal	high
total RBC		•	•†
PCV		•	•†
total WBC	•	•	•
neutrophils	•	•	•
bands		•	•
lymphocytes			
monocytes			
eosinophils			
basophils			
platelets			
fibrinogen			

Urinalysis

	normal	abnormal
color		
blood	•	•†
protein	•	•†
albumin		
glucose		
pH		
specific gravity	•	•†
WBC		
RBC	•	•†
epithelial cells		
bacteria		
casts	•	•†
crystals		

Special Tests

- Cytology of the abdominal fluid is normal or reveals an elevation in protein concentration and WBC.

• Changes caused by the disease itself
•† Changes secondary to dysfunction caused by the disease

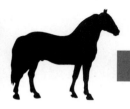

PERITONITIS

Inflammation of the peritoneum can cause fever, abdominal pain, hypovolemic or endotoxic shock, diarrhea, and nasogastric reflux. Causes of septic peritonitis include gastrointestinal perforation, gastrointestinal inflammation or infarction with transmural migration of bacteria, abdominal abscessation, verminous arteritis, septicemia, omphalophlebitis, uterine perforation, complications of abdominal surgery, enterocentesis, complications associated with castration, and penetrating abdominal wounds. Causes of nonseptic peritonitis include gastrointestinal inflammation without transmural migration of bacteria, hemoperitoneum, neoplasia, verminous arteritis, equine viral arteritis, equine infectious anemia, urinary tract perforation, abdominocentesis, and abdominal surgery.

INTERPRETATION OF LABORATORY DATA

PCV may be increased because of hemoconcentration. Serum protein concentration may increase during chronic peritonitis as a result of globulin production or may decrease during acute peritonitis as a result of leakage of large quantities of protein into the peritoneal cavity. When the duration of the inflammation is greater than 48 hours, hyperfibrinogenemia occurs. The acute inflammatory process and/or endotoxemia often results in neutropenia, toxic changes, and a left shift. During chronic inflammation, increased WBC resulting from neutrophilia and nonregenerative anemia are occasionally seen. Poor perfusion due to hypovolemia and endotoxic shock causes metabolic acidosis (decreased total CO_2). Hypovolemia may result in prerenal or renal azotemia (increased SUN and creatinine) or hepatic necrosis (increased SDH and AST). Renal azotemia may be accompanied by isosthenuric specific gravity (1.008 to 1.012), and sometimes blood, casts, and protein in urine sediment. Decreased feed intake causes hypokalemia.

SIGNIFICANT DISEASES TO RULE OUT

♦ Strangulating obstruction causes severe distention of the small or large intestine on rectal examination.
♦ Colitis does not frequently cause changes in the abdominal fluid protein content or WBC concentration.
♦ Abdominal abscessation can sometimes be definitively diagnosed by identification of an abdominal mass via rectal or ultrasonographic examination.

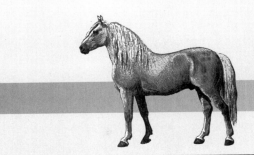

Signs

- ◆ Fever
- ◆ Abdominal pain
- ◆ Hypovolemic and endotoxic shock
- ◆ Diarrhea
- ◆ Nasogastric reflux

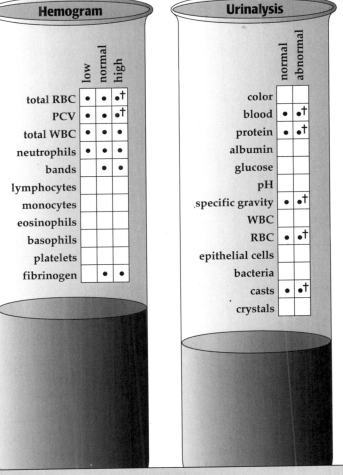

Serum Chemistry

	low	normal	high
CK			
AST		•	•†
SDH		•	•†
GGT			
bile acids			
bilirubin, total			
bilirubin, direct			
protein, total	•	•	•†
albumin	•	•	•†
globulin	•	•	•
SUN		•	•†
creatinine		•	•†
glucose			
Ca			
P			
Na			
K	•†	•	
Cl			
tCO₂	•	•	

Hemogram

	low	normal	high
total RBC	•	•	•†
PCV	•	•	•†
total WBC	•	•	•
neutrophils	•	•	•
bands		•	•
lymphocytes			
monocytes			
eosinophils			
basophils			
platelets			
fibrinogen		•	•

Urinalysis

	normal	abnormal
color		
blood	•	•†
protein	•	•†
albumin		
glucose		
pH		
specific gravity	•	•†
WBC		
RBC	•	•†
epithelial cells		
bacteria		
casts	•	•†
crystals		

Special Tests

- ◆ Abdominal fluid cytology reveals elevation of WBC and protein concentration with or without bacteria and degenerative neutrophils.
- ◆ Microbiology of abdominal fluid sometimes reveals positive culture.

- • Changes caused by the disease itself
- •† Changes secondary to dysfunction caused by the disease

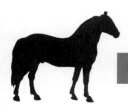

ACUTE COLITIS

Inflammatory conditions of the large intestine can cause acute diarrhea, endotoxemia, and abdominal pain. Causes of acute colitis include *Salmonella* spp., *Ehrlichia risticii* (Potomac horse fever), *Clostridium* spp., parasitism, sand, heavy metal toxicosis, grain overload, and antimicrobial drugs.

INTERPRETATION OF LABORATORY DATA

WBC reveals leukopenia caused by neutropenia, a left shift, toxic changes, and sometimes lymphopenia. Inflammation of the bowel wall may cause mild increases in plasma fibrinogen concentration. Gastrointestinal losses of electrolytes and anorexia lead to hyponatremia, hypochloremia, hypokalemia, and metabolic acidosis (decreased total CO_2). Hypocalcemia is sometimes seen. Metabolic acidosis also results from hypovolemia and endotoxic shock. Elevations of SUN and creatinine frequently result from prerenal azotemia caused by hypovolemia. However, renal azotemia (isosthenuric specific gravity 1.008 to 1.012 with blood, protein, and casts in the urine) occasionally results from tubular necrosis caused by hypovolemia, endotoxemia, and treatment with renal toxic drugs. Hemoconcentration (increased PCV and serum protein) may result from loss of fluid into the intestinal lumen. Protein-losing enteropathy decreases serum protein concentration. However, in the face of hemoconcentration, serum protein concentration may be normal. Stress and endotoxemia may increase the blood glucose concentration; however, the blood glucose concentration decreases during some stages of endotoxemia. Horses with severe endotoxic shock may develop disseminated intravascular coagulopathy, which frequently causes thrombocytopenia.

SIGNIFICANT DISEASES TO RULE OUT

- Nonstrangulating obstruction will cause large intestinal displacement, distention, or impaction palpable via rectal examination.
- Peritonitis elevates plasma fibrinogen (when the duration is greater than 48 hours) and the abdominal fluid protein concentration.

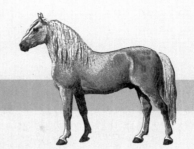

Signs

- ◆ Diarrhea
- ◆ Endotoxemia
- ◆ Abdominal pain

Serum Chemistry

	low	normal	high
CK			
AST			
SDH			
GGT			
bile acids			
bilirubin, total			
bilirubin, direct			
protein, total	•	•	•†
albumin	•	•	•†
globulin	•	•	•†
SUN		•	•†
creatinine		•	•†
glucose	•†	•	•†
Ca	•	•	
P			
Na	•	•	
K	•	•	
Cl	•	•	
tCO₂	•	•	

Hemogram

	low	normal	high
total RBC		•	•†
PCV		•	•†
total WBC	•	•	•
neutrophils	•	•	•
bands		•	•
lymphocytes	•	•	
monocytes			
eosinophils			
basophils			
platelets	•	•	
fibrinogen		•	•

Urinalysis

	normal	abnormal
color		
blood	•	•†
protein	•	•†
albumin		
glucose		
pH		
specific gravity	•	•†
WBC		
RBC	•	•†
epithelial cells		
bacteria		
casts	•	•†
crystals		

Special Tests

- ◆ Abdominal fluid cytology is normal except when bowel inflammation or intestinal wall necrosis elevates protein concentration.
- ◆ Microbiology may reveal culture of *Salmonella* spp. from feces.
- ◆ Serology may reveal increase or decrease in serum IFA antibody titer to *Ehrlichia risticii* over 7 to 10 days.
- ◆ Fecal examination may reveal large quantities of sand or parasites.
- ◆ Toxicology may reveal high concentrations of arsenic in blood or tissues.

- • Changes caused by the disease itself
- •† Changes secondary to dysfunction caused by the disease

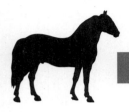

FOAL DIARRHEA

Causes of foal diarrhea include bacteria, viruses, nutrition, parasites, septicemia, intestinal obstruction, peritonitis, and antimicrobial treatment. Diarrhea sometimes occurs during the mare's foal heat as a result of physiologic changes in the foal's digestive tract. Damage to the intestinal mucosa may lead to endotoxemia or septicemia, leading to rapid onset of depression and shock. In contrast to adult horses, foals are prone to developing septicemia concurrent with diarrhea.

INTERPRETATION OF LABORATORY DATA

CBC may indicate endotoxemia or septicemia with a neutropenia and a left shift. Sometimes, chronic intestinal inflammation increases neutrophil count. Hypovolemia reduces glomerular filtration, thereby increasing SUN and creatinine. Prolonged reduction in renal perfusion during endotoxemia and hypovolemia can result in renal azotemia (increased SUN and creatinine concentration, urine specific gravity 1.008 to 1.012, sometimes blood protein or casts in urine sediment). Urine specific gravity is commonly 1.008 to 1.012 in normal foals. Failure of passive transfer or intestinal protein loss may decrease globulin concentration. Hemoconcentration results in increased PCV and RBC. Hemoconcentration concurrent with intestinal losses of protein can result in normal serum protein and albumin concentrations. Hyponatremia results from gastrointestinal and renal (if renal failure develops) losses. Hypokalemia can result from intestinal losses of potassium and decreased food intake. Hypovolemia and intestinal losses of bicarbonate decrease total CO_2 concentration. Hyperkalemia can result from a shift of intracellular potassium to the extracellular space as a result of acidosis.

SIGNIFICANT DISEASES TO RULE OUT

◆ Septicemia can sometimes be confirmed by positive blood cultures.

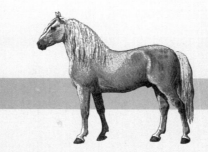

Signs

- Diarrhea
- Depression
- Anorexia
- Endotoxic or hypovolemic shock
- Fever

Serum Chemistry

	low	normal	high
CK			
AST			
SDH			
GGT			
bile acids			
bilirubin, total			
bilirubin, direct			
protein, total	•	•	•†
albumin	•	•	•†
globulin	•	•	
SUN		•	•†
creatinine		•	•†
glucose	•	•	
Ca			
P			
Na	•	•	
K	•	•	•
Cl	•	•	
tCO₂	•	•	

Hemogram

	low	normal	high
total RBC		•	•†
PCV		•	•†
total WBC	•	•	•
neutrophils	•	•	
bands		•	•
lymphocytes			
monocytes			
eosinophils			
basophils			
platelets	·		
fibrinogen			

Urinalysis

	normal	abnormal
color		
blood	•	•†
protein	•	•†
albumin		
glucose		
pH		
specific gravity	•	•
WBC		
RBC	•	•†
epithelial cells		
bacteria		
casts	•	•†
crystals		

Special Tests

- Abdominocentesis is usually normal unless intestinal obstruction or perforation leads to peritonitis.
- Enteritis can lead to septicemia, resulting in positive blood cultures.
- Fecal culture for *Salmonella* can be positive.
- ELISA or latex agglutination test for rotavirus can be positive.

• Changes caused by the disease itself
•† Changes secondary to dysfunction caused by the disease

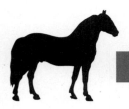

CANTHARIDIN TOXICITY (BLISTER BEETLE)

Toxicity results from ingestion of cantharidin-containing beetles belonging to the family Meloidae. The blister beetles are killed during harvesting of forages (especially alfalfa) and ingested with hay. Clinical signs include abdominal pain, diarrhea, dysuria, and a stiff gait.

INTERPRETATION OF LABORATORY DATA

Hemoconcentration (increased PCV and serum protein), hypocalcemia, and hypomagnesemia are common laboratory findings. Neutropenia with a left shift may be seen as a result of endotoxemia. Alternatively, stress may cause a neutrophilia. Prerenal azotemia is common because of hypovolemia. However, renal azotemia (isosthenuric specific gravity 1.008 to 1.012 with blood, protein, and casts) may also result from tubular necrosis due to the toxin. Hematuria most often results from toxin-induced necrosis of the bladder mucosa. As the disease progresses, decreased serum protein results from urinary and gastrointestinal losses of protein. Hypovolemia and endotoxic shock may lead to metabolic acidosis (decreased total CO_2).

SIGNIFICANT DISEASES TO RULE OUT

- Colitis due to other causes is not accompanied by dysuria resulting from necrosis of the bladder mucosa or profound hypocalcemia and hypomagnesemia.
- Peritonitis elevates the abdominal fluid protein concentration and WBC.

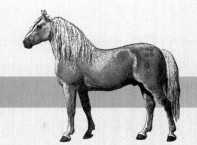

Signs

- ◆ Abdominal pain
- ◆ Diarrhea
- ◆ Dysuria
- ◆ Stiff gait

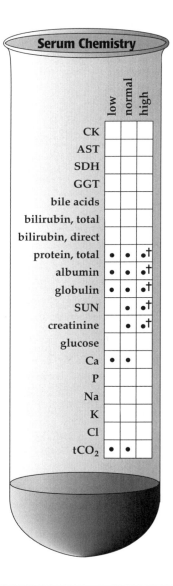

Serum Chemistry

	low	normal	high
CK			
AST			
SDH			
GGT			
bile acids			
bilirubin, total			
bilirubin, direct			
protein, total	•	•	•†
albumin	•	•	•†
globulin	•	•	•†
SUN		•	•†
creatinine		•	•†
glucose			
Ca	•	•	
P			
Na			
K			
Cl			
tCO₂	•	•	

Hemogram

	low	normal	high
total RBC		•	•†
PCV		•	•†
total WBC	•	•	•
neutrophils	•	•	•
bands		•	•
lymphocytes			
monocytes			
eosinophils			
basophils			
platelets			
fibrinogen			

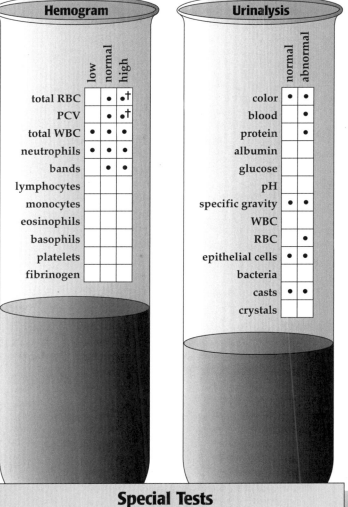

Urinalysis

	normal	abnormal
color	•	•
blood		•
protein		•
albumin		
glucose		
pH		
specific gravity	•	•
WBC		
RBC		•
epithelial cells	•	•
bacteria		
casts	•	•
crystals		

Special Tests

- ◆ Toxicologic examination of urine may reveal cantharidin.
- ◆ Hypomagnesemia frequently accompanies hypocalcemia.

• Changes caused by the disease itself

•† Changes secondary to dysfunction caused by the disease

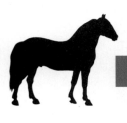

NONSTEROIDAL ANTIINFLAMMATORY DRUG (NSAID) TOXICITY

Mucosal ulcerations of the gingiva, hard palate, tongue, stomach, small intestine, and large intestine can result from NSAID toxicity. A localized right dorsal colitis has also been described in association with this toxicity. Toxicity results from overdose and from treatment with standard dosage regimens. Weight loss, intermittent colic, diarrhea, anorexia, and depression are among the clinical signs.

INTERPRETATION OF LABORATORY DATA

Decreased serum protein concentration and albumin concentration result from exudation of protein into the intestinal lumen. Renal papillary necrosis can cause proteinuria. Leukopenia and neutropenia with a left shift are associated with endotoxemia. Hypokalemia may result from decreased feed intake. Renal or prerenal azotemia may result from arteriolar vasoconstriction by the NSAID. Renal azotemia may result in casts and isosthenuria (specific gravity 1.008 to 1.012).

SIGNIFICANT DISEASES TO RULE OUT

◆ Colitis due to other causes can be confirmed by either culture of *Salmonella* organisms from feces, rising or falling serum antibody titer to *Ehrlichia risticii*, or detection of large amounts of sand in feces.
◆ Nonstrangulating infarction usually elevates the abdominal fluid protein concentration and WBC.
◆ Peritonitis elevates the plasma fibrinogen concentration (if duration is greater than 48 hours), the abdominal fluid protein concentration, and the WBC.

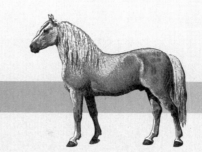

Signs

- ◆ Mucosal ulcerations
- ◆ Weight loss
- ◆ Abdominal pain
- ◆ Diarrhea
- ◆ Endotoxic and hypovolemic shock

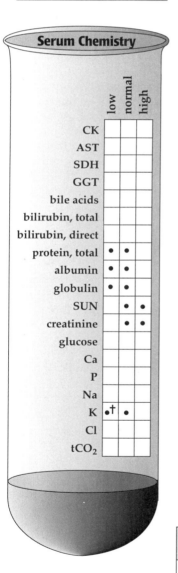

Serum Chemistry

	low	normal	high
CK			
AST			
SDH			
GGT			
bile acids			
bilirubin, total			
bilirubin, direct			
protein, total	•	•	
albumin	•	•	
globulin	•	•	
SUN		•	•
creatinine		•	•
glucose			
Ca			
P			
Na			
K	•†	•	
Cl			
tCO$_2$			

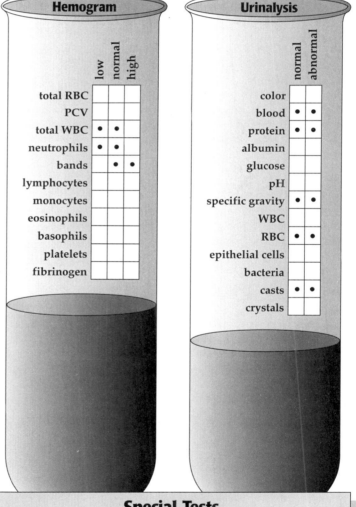

Hemogram

	low	normal	high
total RBC			
PCV			
total WBC	•	•	
neutrophils	•	•	
bands		•	•
lymphocytes			
monocytes			
eosinophils			
basophils			
platelets			
fibrinogen			

Urinalysis

	normal	abnormal
color		
blood	•	•
protein	•	•
albumin		
glucose		
pH		
specific gravity	•	•
WBC		
RBC	•	•
epithelial cells		
bacteria		
casts	•	•
crystals		

Special Tests

- ◆ Cytology of the abdominal fluid rarely reveals increased abdominal fluid protein concentration and WBC count.

• Changes caused by the disease itself

•† Changes secondary to dysfunction caused by the disease

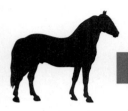

INTESTINAL NEOPLASIA

Lymphosarcoma, the most common intestinal neoplasm, affects horses of all ages and causes diffuse infiltration of the intestinal wall by tumor cells. Carbohydrate malabsorption and weight loss are the most common sequelae. Diarrhea results when the disease progresses to involve the large intestine. Adenocarcinoma and leiomyosarcoma occur rarely in the equine intestine.

INTERPRETATION OF LABORATORY DATA

Nonregenerative anemia results from neoplastic disease. Rarely, decreased serum protein concentration results from protein exudation into the intestinal tract. Chronic inflammation more often causes increased serum protein concentration as a result of increased globulin concentration. Increased fibrinogen concentration, neutrophilia, and leukocytosis also may accompany the inflammatory reaction.

SIGNIFICANT DISEASES TO RULE OUT

- ◆ Parasitism usually is confirmed by response to larvacidal anthelmintic therapy.
- ◆ Granulomatous enteritis can only be confirmed by demonstration of granulomatous infiltration of a biopsy of the intestinal wall.
- ◆ Abdominal abscessation elevates the abdominal fluid protein concentration and WBC. In some cases an abdominal mass is palpable per rectal examination or visible via ultrasonographic examination.

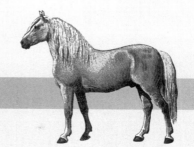

Signs

- Weight loss
- Diarrhea
- Abdominal pain

Serum Chemistry

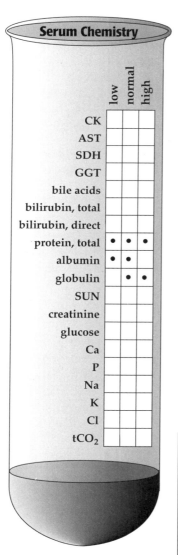

	low	normal	high
CK			
AST			
SDH			
GGT			
bile acids			
bilirubin, total			
bilirubin, direct			
protein, total	•	•	•
albumin	•	•	
globulin		•	•
SUN			
creatinine			
glucose			
Ca			
P			
Na			
K			
Cl			
tCO$_2$			

Hemogram

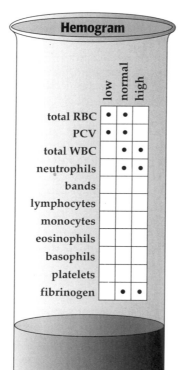

	low	normal	high
total RBC	•	•	
PCV	•	•	
total WBC		•	•
neutrophils		•	•
bands			
lymphocytes			
monocytes			
eosinophils			
basophils			
platelets			
fibrinogen		•	•

Urinalysis

	normal	abnormal
color		
blood		
protein		
albumin		
glucose		
pH		
specific gravity		
WBC		
RBC		
epithelial cells		
bacteria		
casts		
crystals		

Special Tests

- Abdominal fluid cytology rarely reveals neoplastic cells.
- Carbohydrate absorption tests sometimes reveal glucose and xylose malabsorption.
- Protein electrophoresis usually reveals polyclonal gammopathy or less commonly monoclonal gammopathy.
- Histopathology reveals neoplastic infiltration of intestinal wall or lymph node.

- • Changes caused by the disease itself
- •† Changes secondary to dysfunction caused by the disease

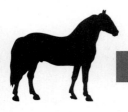

PARASITISM

Infestations with large (*Strongylus vulgaris* and *Triodontophorus*) and small strongyles (*Cyathostomum* and related genera) are among the most common causes of intestinal disease in horses. Weight loss, abdominal pain, and/or diarrhea are common clinical signs.

INTERPRETATION OF LABORATORY DATA

Nonregenerative anemia and hyperglobulinemia often result from chronic intestinal inflammation due to parasitism. Regenerative anemia and decreased serum protein concentration occasionally result from intestinal blood loss. Horses do not commonly develop eosinophilia due to parasitism. Severe illness may decrease feed and water intake, leading to hemoconcentration, prerenal azotemia, and hypokalemia. Intestinal or colonic wall inflammation (colitis) can allow absorption of endotoxin, causing neutropenia, a left shift, toxic changes, increased plasma fibrinogen, and intestinal protein loss.

SIGNIFICANT DISEASES TO RULE OUT

◆ Granulomatous enteritis can only be confirmed by demonstration of granulomatous infiltration of a biopsy of the intestinal wall.
◆ Abdominal abscessation causes an elevation in abdominal fluid protein concentration and WBC and an elevation in plasma fibrinogen concentration.
◆ Intestinal neoplasia is confirmed by finding neoplastic infiltration of the intestinal wall or peripheral lymph node.

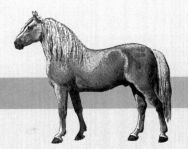

Signs

- ◆ Weight loss
- ◆ Abdominal pain
- ◆ Diarrhea

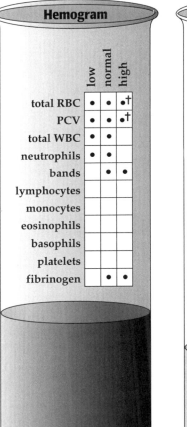

Serum Chemistry

	low	normal	high
CK			
AST			
SDH			
GGT			
bile acids			
bilirubin, total			
bilirubin, direct			
protein, total	•	•	•†
albumin	•	•	
globulin	•	•	•
SUN		•	•†
creatinine		•	•†
glucose			
Ca			
P			
Na			
K	•†	•	
Cl			
tCO$_2$			

Hemogram

	low	normal	high
total RBC	•	•	•†
PCV	•	•	•†
total WBC	•	•	
neutrophils	•	•	
bands		•	•
lymphocytes			
monocytes			
eosinophils			
basophils			
platelets			
fibrinogen		•	•

Urinalysis

	normal	abnormal
color		
blood		
protein		
albumin		
glucose		
pH		
specific gravity		
WBC		
RBC		
epithelial cells		
bacteria		
casts		
crystals		

Special Tests

- ◆ Parasitology may reveal increased numbers of ova or may be negative for parasite ova when disease is due to larval stages.
- ◆ Abdominal fluid cytology may be normal or reveal a mild increase in WBC with or without eosinophils.
- ◆ D-xylose or glucose test may reveal malabsorption.

- • Changes caused by the disease itself
- •† Changes secondary to dysfunction caused by the disease

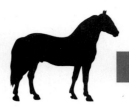

INTRAABDOMINAL ABSCESSATION

Abscessation of abdominal lymph nodes results from dissemination of bacteria via the bloodstream or lymphatic system. Perforation of the intestine or penetration of the abdominal wall may result in local peritonitis and abscess formation. Abdominal abscessation may cause weight loss, fever, and abdominal pain. An abdominal mass is sometimes palpable via rectal examination. Specific etiologies include *Streptococcus equi* and *zooepidemicus*, *Rhodococcus equi*, gram-negative bacteria, and anaerobic bacteria.

INTERPRETATION OF LABORATORY DATA

The chronic septic inflammation increases the plasma fibrinogen concentration and serum globulin concentration and causes nonregenerative anemia. Peripheral WBC and neutrophil count are less commonly increased.

SIGNIFICANT DISEASES TO RULE OUT

- Parasitism responds to larvacidal anthelmintic therapy.
- Granulomatous enteritis decreases serum protein concentration and causes granulomatous infiltration of the intestinal wall.
- Intestinal neoplasia causes neoplastic infiltration of intestinal wall or peripheral lymph node.

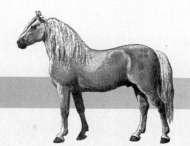

Signs

- Weight loss
- Fever
- Abdominal pain

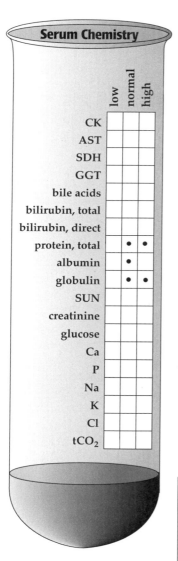

Serum Chemistry

	low	normal	high
CK			
AST			
SDH			
GGT			
bile acids			
bilirubin, total			
bilirubin, direct			
protein, total		•	•
albumin		•	
globulin		•	•
SUN			
creatinine			
glucose			
Ca			
P			
Na			
K			
Cl			
tCO$_2$			

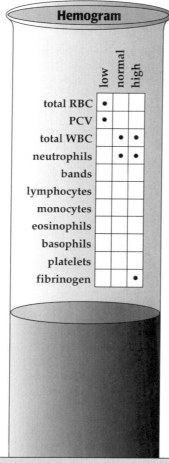

Hemogram

	low	normal	high
total RBC	•		
PCV	•		
total WBC		•	•
neutrophils		•	•
bands			
lymphocytes			
monocytes			
eosinophils			
basophils			
platelets			
fibrinogen			•

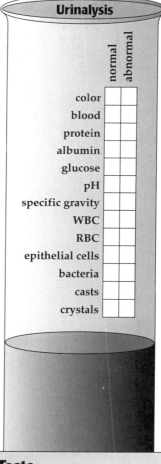

Urinalysis

	normal	abnormal
color		
blood		
protein		
albumin		
glucose		
pH		
specific gravity		
WBC		
RBC		
epithelial cells		
bacteria		
casts		
crystals		

Special Tests

- Abdominal fluid cytology reveals increased WBC and protein concentration with bacteria rarely seen.
- Microbiology of peritoneal fluid sometimes reveals bacteria.
- Ultrasonography of abdomen occasionally demonstrates the abscess.

• Changes caused by the disease itself
•† Changes secondary to dysfunction caused by the disease

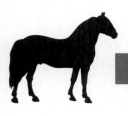

GRANULOMATOUS, EOSINOPHILIC, LYMPHOCYTIC, AND BASOPHILIC ENTERITIS

Idiopathic granulomatous, eosinophilic, basophilic, or lymphocytic infiltration of the small intestinal wall may result in malabsorption and weight loss. Later in the disease process, involvement of the large intestine causes diarrhea. Hypoproteinemia may lead to dependent edema.

INTERPRETATION OF LABORATORY DATA

The most common laboratory findings are decreased serum protein and globulin concentrations as a result of exudation into the intestinal lumen. Nonregenerative anemia is often seen as a result of the chronic inflammation.

SIGNIFICANT DISEASES TO RULE OUT

- ◆ Intestinal neoplasia is diagnosed by neoplastic infiltration of intestinal wall or peripheral lymph node.
- ◆ Parasitism usually responds to larvacidal anthelmintic therapy.
- ◆ Abdominal abscessation elevates the abdominal fluid protein concentration and WBC. An abdominal mass may be palpable via rectal examination or visible on ultrasonographic examination.
- ◆ Chronic liver disease can lead to weight loss with decreased serum albumin concentration. Liver disease also increases bile acids, bilirubin, and serum activity of SDH and GGT.

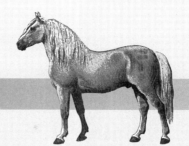

Signs

- ◆ Weight loss
- ◆ Diarrhea
- ◆ Rarely colic

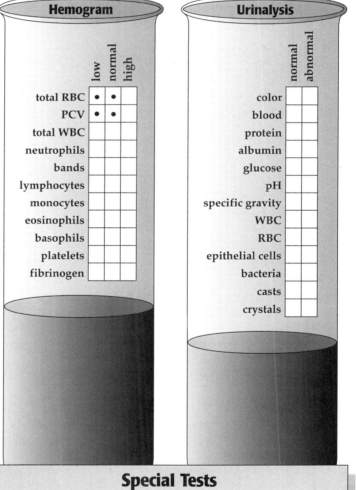

Serum Chemistry

	low	normal	high
CK			
AST			
SDH			
GGT			
bile acids			
bilirubin, total			
bilirubin, direct			
protein, total	•	•	
albumin	•	•	
globulin	•	•	
SUN			
creatinine			
glucose			
Ca			
P			
Na			
K			
Cl			
tCO$_2$			

Hemogram

	low	normal	high
total RBC	•	•	
PCV	•	•	
total WBC			
neutrophils			
bands			
lymphocytes			
monocytes			
eosinophils			
basophils			
platelets			
fibrinogen			

Urinalysis

	normal	abnormal
color		
blood		
protein		
albumin		
glucose		
pH		
specific gravity		
WBC		
RBC		
epithelial cells		
bacteria		
casts		
crystals		

Special Tests

- ◆ Carbohydrate absorption tests often reveal xylose and glucose malabsorption.
- ◆ Histopathology of intestinal biopsy reveals granulomatous, eosinophilic, basophilic, or lymphocytic infiltration of the intestinal wall.

• Changes caused by the disease itself

•† Changes secondary to dysfunction caused by the disease

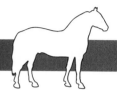

SECTION SEVEN

Musculoskeletal Diseases

Septic arthritis and osteomyelitis

Immune-mediated polysynovitis

Lyme borreliosis

Exertional rhabdomyolysis

Nutritional myodegeneration

Bacterial myonecrosis

Toxic myopathy

Hyperkalemic periodic paralysis

Hypocalcemia

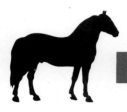

SEPTIC ARTHRITIS AND OSTEOMYELITIS

Bacterial synovitis with or without bone infection occurs as a sequela to bacteremia, trauma, arthrocentesis, or surgery. Clinical signs include fever, lameness, swelling, depression, and difficulty rising. Bacterial isolates include *E. coli*, *Klebsiella* sp., streptococci, *Actinobacillus equuli*, and *Rhodococcus equi*. Fungal arthritis (esp. *Candida* sp.) has been infrequently diagnosed as a sequela to systemic infection. Prognosis is always guarded and depends on the extent of bone, joint, and cartilage damage and the ability to remove the infection. Involvement of other organs is common in neonates with failure of passive transfer.

INTERPRETATION OF LABORATORY DATA

Peripheral leukocyte count may be increased because of neutrophilia resulting from chronic inflammation. Concurrent bacteremia often causes leukopenia, neutropenia, and a left shift. Inflammation increases the plasma fibrinogen concentration; however, early in the disease the fibrinogen may be normal. Chronic inflammation may increase the globulin concentration. A nonregenerative anemia sometimes is seen in chronic cases.

SIGNIFICANT DISEASES TO RULE OUT

◆ Trauma sometimes causes no distinguishing findings. Trauma only causes mild increases in synovial fluid cell count and protein.
◆ Immune-mediated polysynovitis is sometimes diagnosed based on failure to identify causative infectious agents. Staining for immune complexes in synovial membranes has not been well validated in horses; however, characteristic findings on histopathologic examination of synovial biopsies are of diagnostic significance. Horses with immune-mediated polysynovitis present with joint distention, but are usually not lame.

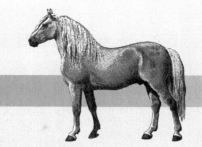

Signs

- ◆ Fever
- ◆ Lameness
- ◆ Swelling
- ◆ Heat
- ◆ Depression
- ◆ Difficulty rising

Serum Chemistry

	low	normal	high
CK			
AST			
SDH			
GGT			
bile acids			
bilirubin, total			
bilirubin, direct			
protein, total		•	•
albumin		•	
globulin		•	•
SUN			
creatinine			
glucose			
Ca			
P			
Na			
K			
Cl			
tCO$_2$			

Hemogram

	low	normal	high
total RBC	•	•	
PCV	•	•	
total WBC		•	•
neutrophils		•	•
bands		•	•
lymphocytes			
monocytes			
eosinophils			
basophils			
platelets			
fibrinogen		•	•

Urinalysis

	normal	abnormal
color		
blood		
protein		
albumin		
glucose		
pH		
specific gravity		
WBC		
RBC		
epithelial cells		
bacteria		
casts		
crystals		

Special Tests

- ◆ Radiographs may reveal arthritis or osteomyelitis.
- ◆ Synovial fluid cytology may reveal increased neutrophil numbers and increased cell count.
- ◆ Synovial fluid or biopsy culture may reveal the causative agent and neutrophilic inflammation.
- ◆ Serum immunoglobulin concentration (ELISA) may be decreased in foals.

• Changes caused by the disease itself
•† Changes secondary to dysfunction caused by the disease

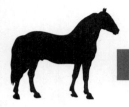

Immune-Mediated Polysynovitis

Synovial effusions in multiple joints and mild lameness in multiple limbs have been observed in foals and rarely in adult horses. Immune-mediated synovitis results from immunoglobulin G deposition in the synovium. Immune complexes formed as a result of a nonarticular focus of infection (most commonly pneumonia, especially due to *Rhodococcus equi*) are deposited into the synovium. Alternatively, immunogenic bacterial byproducts may localize in the synovium and attract immunoglobulin. These immune complexes stimulate a lymphocytic plasmacytic synovitis. Rarely, a specific immune-mediated systemic syndrome (lupus erythematosus–like polysynovitis) has been described in horses. In addition to multiple joint swellings and stiffness, clinical signs related to the focus of infection may be seen.

Interpretation of Laboratory Data

The nonarticular focus of infection often results in peripheral neutrophilia and hyperfibrinogenemia. White blood cell count in the synovial fluid sometimes is mildly increased (up to 15,000 cells/ml). Rheumatoid factor titers, antinuclear antibody titers, lupus erythematosus cell preparations, and Coombs' test are usually negative. However, these tests could be positive as a result of nonspecific mechanisms or as a result of lupus erythematosus–like disease.

Significant Diseases to Rule Out

◆ Septic arthritis causes severe joint swelling and severe lameness. Synovial fluid cytology reveals cell counts in excess of 15,000 cells/ml. Synovial biopsy reveals neutrophilic synovitis without immune complex deposition. Synovial fluid and biopsy culture may reveal the infectious organism.

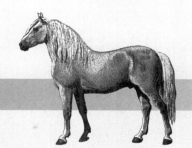

Signs

- ◆ Synovial effusions in multiple joints
- ◆ Mild lameness

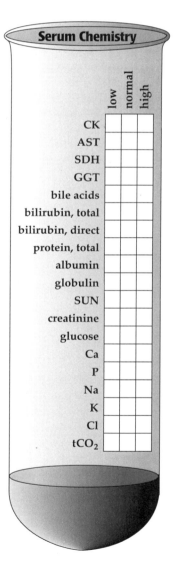

Serum Chemistry

	low	normal	high
CK			
AST			
SDH			
GGT			
bile acids			
bilirubin, total			
bilirubin, direct			
protein, total			
albumin			
globulin			
SUN			
creatinine			
glucose			
Ca			
P			
Na			
K			
Cl			
tCO$_2$			

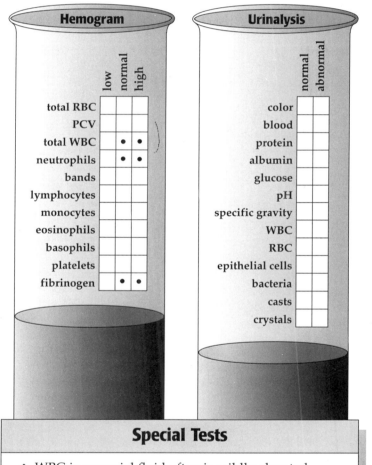

Hemogram

	low	normal	high
total RBC			
PCV			
total WBC		●	●
neutrophils		●	●
bands			
lymphocytes			
monocytes			
eosinophils			
basophils			
platelets			
fibrinogen		●	●

Urinalysis

	normal	abnormal
color		
blood		
protein		
albumin		
glucose		
pH		
specific gravity		
WBC		
RBC		
epithelial cells		
bacteria		
casts		
crystals		

Special Tests

- ◆ WBC in synovial fluid often is mildly elevated.
- ◆ Cultures of synovial fluid and synovial biopsy are negative.
- ◆ Histologic examination of synovial biopsy reveals lymphocytic plasmacytic synovitis.
- ◆ Immune complexes may be demonstrated with fluorescent antibody staining of the synovium. However, this test may be difficult to evaluate in horses, because of inadequate validation.

- ● Changes caused by the disease itself
- ●† Changes secondary to dysfunction caused by the disease

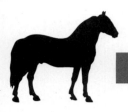

LYME BORRELIOSIS

Lyme disease is a complex and multi-systemic disease caused by a spirochete organism, *Borrelia burgdorferi*. It most often presents as arthritis. Encephalitis has been recognized, but skin lesions have not been reported in the horse. In addition to arthritis in single or multiple joints, clinical signs may include lethargy, fever, and anterior uveitis.

INTERPRETATION OF LABORATORY DATA

Synovial fluid analysis demonstrates inflammation with increased numbers of neutrophils; histopathology of synovial membrane reveals a mononuclear infiltrate. The CBC reflects a neutrophilic leukocytosis. Antibody titers are commonly used in diagnosis, but must be interpreted with caution since concentrations do not distinguish between clinical cases and inapparent infections. Culture of *Borrelia burgdorferi* or identifying the spirochete microscopically is definitive, but difficult.

SIGNIFICANT DISEASES TO RULE OUT

- Any other cause of arthritis must be included in the differential diagnosis.
- Trauma may be diagnosed by history and physical examination, and causes only mild increases in synovial fluid cell count and protein.
- Septic arthritis causes severe joint swelling and lameness. Synovial fluid cytology reveals cell counts in excess of 15,000 cells/µl. Synovial biopsy reveals neutrophilic synovitis without immune complex deposition. Synovial fluid and biopsy culture may reveal the infectious organism.
- Immune-mediated polysynovitis is sometimes diagnosed based on failure to identify causative infectious agents. Staining for immune complexes in synovial membranes has not been well validated in horses. Horses with immune-mediated polysynovitis present with joint distention, but are usually not lame.

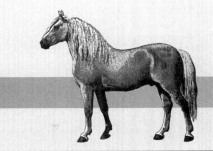

Signs

- ◆ Arthritis in single or multiple joints
- ◆ Anterior uveitis
- ◆ Lethargy
- ◆ Fever

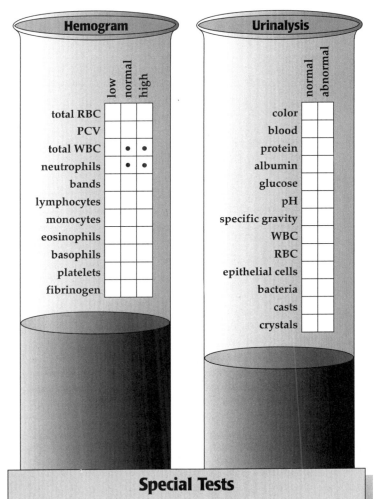

Serum Chemistry

	low	normal	high
CK			
AST			
SDH			
GGT			
bile acids			
bilirubin, total			
bilirubin, direct			
protein, total			
albumin			
globulin			
SUN			
creatinine			
glucose			
Ca			
P			
Na			
K			
Cl			
tCO$_2$			

Hemogram

	low	normal	high
total RBC			
PCV			
total WBC		•	•
neutrophils		•	•
bands			
lymphocytes			
monocytes			
eosinophils			
basophils			
platelets			
fibrinogen			

Urinalysis

	normal	abnormal
color		
blood		
protein		
albumin		
glucose		
pH		
specific gravity		
WBC		
RBC		
epithelial cells		
bacteria		
casts		
crystals		

Special Tests

- ◆ Synovial fluid analysis may reveal increased protein and neutrophils.
- ◆ Synovial biopsy specimens show a mononuclear cell infiltrate and villous hypertrophy.
- ◆ Culture and identification or antibody titers may be positive for *Borrelia*.

- • Changes caused by the disease itself
- •† Changes secondary to dysfunction caused by the disease

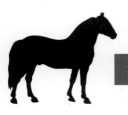

EXERTIONAL RHABDOMYOLYSIS

Exertional rhabdomyolysis is muscle dysfunction occurring after exercise, resulting in gait abnormalities (stiffness), muscle pain, tachycardia, tachypnea, sweating, myoglobinuria, and sometimes recumbency. The disease is sometimes associated with changes in management practices and training schedule, inadequate preparation for competition, metabolic imbalances (e.g., hypokalemia), or heritable traits.

INTERPRETATION OF LABORATORY DATA

Serum activity of CK and AST is usually increased in horses with exertional rhabdomyolysis. Serum activity of CK decreases rapidly with resolution of myonecrosis, owing to a short half-life, while activity of AST remains increased for several days. Although hypovolemia and metabolic acidosis (decreased total CO_2) sometimes develop in severe cases, hemoconcentration (increased PCV and total serum protein), hypochloremic metabolic alkalosis, and hypocalcemia are more common abnormalities. Hypokalemia is common because of reduced potassium intake and loss through excessive sweating. Myoglobinuria is common in severe cases. SUN and creatinine may be increased because of hypovolemia or tubular damage by myoglobin. When renal failure develops, urine specific gravity is in the isosthenuric range. Casts may appear in the urinary sediment because of tubular damage.

SIGNIFICANT DISEASES TO RULE OUT

◆ Laminitis will only cause slight increases in serum activity of CK and AST. The pain can be localized to the foot by assessing the response to posterior digital nerve block.
◆ Abdominal pain will cause only slight increases in serum activity of CK and AST. The muscles are not painful, but the animal may show signs of gastrointestinal disease, such as nasogastric reflux, abnormal feces, or abnormal rectal examination.

Signs

- ◆ Stiffness
- ◆ Pain
- ◆ Tachycardia
- ◆ Tachypnea
- ◆ Sweating
- ◆ Myoglobinuria
- ◆ Recumbency

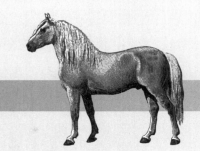

Serum Chemistry

	low	normal	high
CK			•
AST			•
SDH			
GGT			
bile acids			
bilirubin, total			
bilirubin, direct			
protein, total			•
albumin			•
globulin			•
SUN		•	•
creatinine		•	•
glucose			
Ca	•	•	
P			
Na			
K	•	•	
Cl	•	•	
tCO_2	•	•	•

Hemogram

	low	normal	high
total RBC		•	•†
PCV	•		•†
total WBC			
neutrophils			
bands			
lymphocytes			
monocytes			
eosinophils			
basophils			
platelets			
fibrinogen			

Urinalysis

	normal	abnormal
color		•
blood		•
protein		•
albumin		
glucose		
pH		
specific gravity	•	•
WBC		
RBC	•	•
epithelial cells		
bacteria		
casts	•	•
crystals		

Special Tests

- ◆ Myoglobinuria can be differentiated from hemoglobinuria by absence of hemoglobin in plasma or failure to precipitate after addition of ammonium sulfate.
- ◆ Fractional urinary excretion of potassium may be decreased in horse with potassium depletion.
- ◆ Submaximal exercise challenge test may be used to demonstrate muscle damage in subclinical cases.

• Changes caused by the disease itself

•† Changes secondary to dysfunction caused by the disease

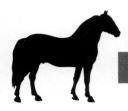

NUTRITIONAL MYODEGENERATION

This is an acute myodegenerative disease of cardiac and skeletal muscle caused by dietary deficiency of vitamin E and selenium. Nutritional myodegeneration occurs mostly in rapidly growing foals but has been suspected in adult horses. The skeletal form is characterized by muscular weakness or stiffness. Animals may be unable to stand or able to stand for only a few minutes. Supporting muscle groups may be swollen, painful, and hard. Involvement of the diaphragm and intercostal muscles may result in respiratory distress. Myoglobinuria may result in brown discoloration of the urine. Involvement of the muscle of the tongue or pharynx may result in dysphagia. Myocardial disease may result in syncope, tachycardia, dependent edema, and jugular pulsation.

INTERPRETATION OF LABORATORY DATA

Skeletal muscle damage will elevate serum activity of CK and AST. Hyperkalemia, hyponatremia, and hypochloremia have been reported. Myoglobinuria can result in a positive urine dipstick test for blood. SUN and creatinine may be increased as a result of hypovolemia or tubular damage by myoglobin. Casts, blood, and/or protein may occur in the urinary sediment. When renal failure occurs, urine specific gravity is in the isosthenuric range.

SIGNIFICANT DISEASES TO RULE OUT

- Laminitis will only cause slight increases in serum activity of CK and AST. The pain can be localized to the foot by assessing the response to posterior digital nerve block.
- Abdominal pain will cause only slight increases in serum activity of CK and AST. The muscles are not painful, but the animal may show signs of gastrointestinal disease, such as nasogastric reflux, abnormal feces, or abnormal rectal examination.
- Botulism may also result in dysphagia and recumbency due to weakness. CK and AST are only mildly elevated; severe generalized muscular weakness is apparent.

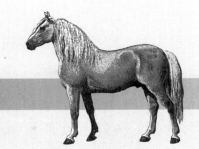

Signs

- ◆ Muscular weakness or stiffness
- ◆ Myoglobimuria

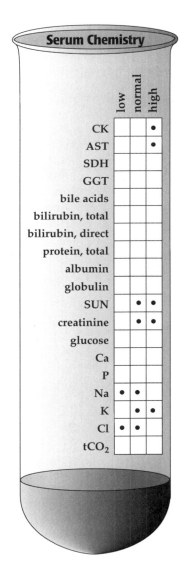

Serum Chemistry

	low	normal	high
CK			•
AST			•
SDH			
GGT			
bile acids			
bilirubin, total			
bilirubin, direct			
protein, total			
albumin			
globulin			
SUN		•	•
creatinine		•	•
glucose			
Ca			
P			
Na	•	•	
K		•	•
Cl	•	•	
tCO$_2$			

Hemogram

	low	normal	high
total RBC			
PCV			
total WBC			
neutrophils			
bands			
lymphocytes			
monocytes			
eosinophils			
basophils			
platelets			
fibrinogen			

Urinalysis

	normal	abnormal
color	•	•
blood	•	•
protein	•	•
albumin		
glucose		
pH		
specific gravity	•	•
WBC		
RBC	•	•
epithelial cells		
bacteria		
casts	•	•
crystals		

Special Tests

- ◆ Plasma concentrations of vitamin E and selenium may be decreased. Decreased activity of selenium-dependent glutathione peroxidase in RBC.

• Changes caused by the disease itself
•† Changes secondary to dysfunction caused by the disease

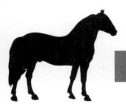

BACTERIAL MYONECROSIS

Wounds that lead to bacterial infection of muscle groups cause muscle necrosis. Puncture wounds, including injections, are the most common predisposing injuries. Fever, anorexia, depression, and tachycardia are common clinical signs. The skin over the affected muscle may become hot and discolored. Crepitation may be palpable. Skin necrosis may lead to sanguineous or purulent drainage. *Clostridium* sp. are among the most common agents causing myonecrosis in horses. Trauma may lead to deposition of aerobic bacteria or *Clostridium* spores. If the conditions within the muscle are suitable, the *Clostridium* spores undergo conversion into the vegetative, toxin-producing form of the organism.

INTERPRETATION OF LABORATORY DATA

Elevations in the serum activity of CK and AST are common. Neutropenia (due to toxemia) or neutrophilia (stress) may cause a leukopenia or leukocytosis, respectively. Toxemia may increase the concentration of band neutrophils. Hypovolemia and toxemia cause hemoconcentration and prerenal azotemia. After 48 hours, plasma fibrinogen concentration may be increased in response to inflammation.

SIGNIFICANT DISEASES TO RULE OUT

◆ Exertional myopathy affects many groups of muscles and is related to exercise.

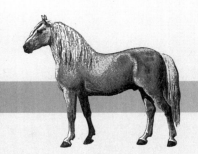

Signs

- ◆ Fever
- ◆ Anorexia
- ◆ Depression
- ◆ Tachycardia
- ◆ Heat
- ◆ Swelling
- ◆ Pain
- ◆ Crepitation

Serum Chemistry

	low	normal	high
CK			•
AST			•
SDH			
GGT			
bile acids			
bilirubin, total			
bilirubin, direct			
protein, total			
albumin			
globulin			
SUN		•	•†
creatinine		•	•†
glucose			
Ca			
P			
Na			
K			
Cl			
tCO$_2$			

Hemogram

	low	normal	high
total RBC			•†
PCV			•†
total WBC	•	•	•
neutrophils	•	•	•
bands		•	•
lymphocytes			
monocytes			
eosinophils			
basophils			
platelets			
fibrinogen		•	•

Urinalysis

	normal	abnormal
color		
blood		
protein		
albumin		
glucose		
pH		
specific gravity		
WBC		
RBC		
epithelial cells		
bacteria		
casts		
crystals		

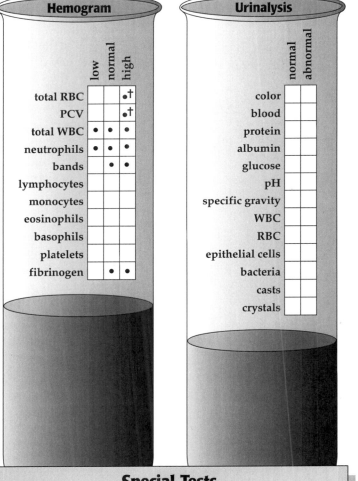

Special Tests

- ◆ Microscopic examination or anaerobic culture of a biopsy or aspirate of the affected muscle may reveal the clostridial organisms.
- ◆ Histopathologic examination of muscle biopsy reveals severe myonecrosis.

• Changes caused by the disease itself
•† Changes secondary to dysfunction caused by the disease

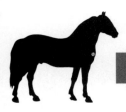

TOXIC MYOPATHY

Horses are very sensitive to the toxic effects of gossypol and the iono-phore antimicrobials (e.g., monensin) commonly used as feed additives in cattle. Castor bean (*Cassia* sp.) ingestion is an uncommon cause of muscle necrosis. In addition, the botulinum C2 toxin causes muscle cell damage and increases in AST and CK. Clinical signs of toxic myopathy include restlessness, colic, anorexia, sweating, reluctance to move, muscle trembling, pyrexia, ataxia, tachycardia, irregular cardiac rhythms, cyanotic mucous membranes, venous distention, jugular distention and pulsation, peripheral edema, murmurs, and acute death. Generalized weakness is the predominant clinical sign of botulism. Ionophore toxicity may also cause nephritis and hepatitis.

INTERPRETATION OF LABORATORY DATA

Packed cell volume, RBC, and protein are increased as a result of hemo-concentration. Elevations of SUN and creatinine may result from pre-renal azotemia or be due to renal necrosis by the toxin. Isosthenuria, hematuria, and urinary casts frequently occur when the ionophores cause renal azotemia. Hepatic damage by the ionophores may cause elevations of bilirubin, bile acids, and the serum activity of AST, SDH, and GGT. Hypocalcemia and hypokalemia are common in the first 24 hours after intoxication with ionophores, but then return to normal. Elevations of serum activity of AST and the cardiac and skeletal isoenzymes of CK are common. However, in chronic cases, the activities of these enzymes may have returned to normal.

DISEASES TO RULE OUT

◆ Exertional myopathy is related to exercise.
◆ Bacterial myonecrosis leads to more severe necrosis of local groups of muscles. Biopsy often will reveal the organism.

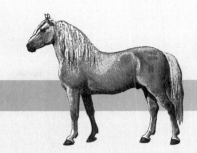

Signs

- Restlessness
- Colic
- Anorexia
- Sweating
- Reluctance to move
- Muscle trembling
- Pyrexia
- Ataxia
- Tachycardia
- Irregular cardiac rhythms
- Cyanotic membranes
- Venous distention
- Edema
- Murmurs
- Acute death

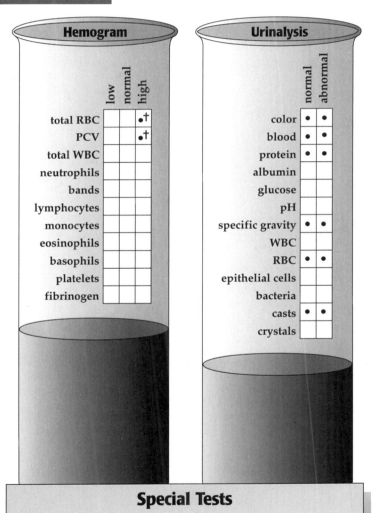

Serum Chemistry

	low	normal	high
CK		•	•
AST		•	•
SDH		•	•
GGT		•	•
bile acids		•	•
bilirubin, total		•	•
bilirubin, direct		•	•
protein, total		•	•†
albumin		•	•†
globulin		•	•†
SUN		•	•
creatinine		•	•
glucose			
Ca	•	•	
P			
Na			
K	•	•	
Cl			
tCO₂			

Hemogram

	low	normal	high
total RBC			•†
PCV			•†
total WBC			
neutrophils			
bands			
lymphocytes			
monocytes			
eosinophils			
basophils			
platelets			
fibrinogen			

Urinalysis

	normal	abnormal
color	•	•
blood	•	•
protein	•	•
albumin		
glucose		
pH		
specific gravity	•	•
WBC		
RBC	•	•
epithelial cells		
bacteria		
casts	•	•
crystals		

Special Tests

- Characteristic lesions will be identified on post-mortem examination.
- Ionophores or gossypol may be detected in feed or intestinal contents.
- CKMB isoenzyme may be increased.

• Changes caused by the disease itself

•† Changes secondary to dysfunction caused by the disease

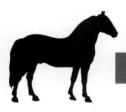

HYPERKALEMIC PERIODIC PARALYSIS

Hyperkalemic periodic paralysis appears to be a biochemical disease of muscle in which there are unpredictable, intermittent, abnormal fluxes of cellular ions (most notably potassium), which last 15 to 60 minutes. This is a familial disease affecting pure and part quarter horses. Clinical signs usually become apparent between 2 and 3 years of age. These fluxes result in transient muscular weakness, muscle fasciculations, third eyelid prolapse, and sweating. Dysphagia also has been associated with periodic hyperkalemia. No abnormalities are apparent between episodes. Horses occasionally die during an episode.

INTERPRETATION OF LABORATORY DATA

Serum potassium concentration is usually but not always increased during clinical manifestation of the disease. Serum activity of CK and creatinine is sometimes slightly increased.

SIGNIFICANT DISEASES TO RULE OUT

◆ Syncope due to cardiac disease will result in electrocardiographic evidence of arrhythmias and/or echocardiographic evidence of cardiac dilation and decreased function.
◆ Hypocalcemia is diagnosed by finding decreased serum calcium concentration.
◆ Tetanus causes persistent clinical signs and is often accompanied by history of a wound.

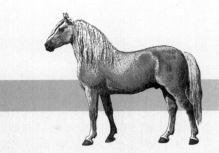

Signs

- ◆ Transient muscular weakness
- ◆ Muscle fasciculations
- ◆ Third eyelid prolapse
- ◆ Sweating

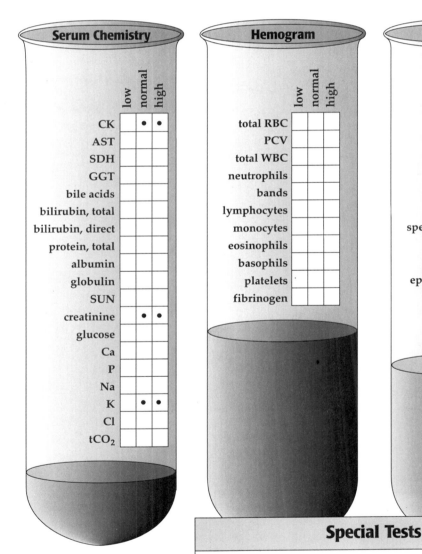

Serum Chemistry

	low	normal	high
CK		•	•
AST			
SDH			
GGT			
bile acids			
bilirubin, total			
bilirubin, direct			
protein, total			
albumin			
globulin			
SUN			
creatinine		•	•
glucose			
Ca			
P			
Na			
K		•	•
Cl			
tCO_2			

Hemogram

	low	normal	high
total RBC			
PCV			
total WBC			
neutrophils			
bands			
lymphocytes			
monocytes			
eosinophils			
basophils			
platelets			
fibrinogen			

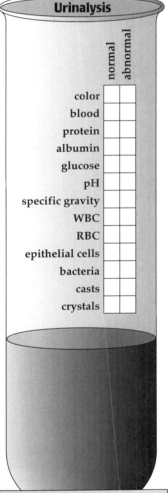

Urinalysis

	normal	abnormal
color		
blood		
protein		
albumin		
glucose		
pH		
specific gravity		
WBC		
RBC		
epithelial cells		
bacteria		
casts		
crystals		

Special Tests

- ◆ Genetic (Veterinary genetics laboratory, University of California, Davis, Calif.) and electromyographic testing aid with diagnosis.

- • Changes caused by the disease itself
- •† Changes secondary to dysfunction caused by the disease

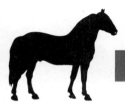

HYPOCALCEMIA

Decreased serum calcium can be caused by gastrointestinal disease, renal disease, lactation, or ingestion of cantharidin (blister beetles). Ionized calcium is responsible for normal membrane function. Clinical signs include increased muscle tone, stiffness, trismus, sweating, and muscle fasciculations. Severe cases can progress to incoordination, recumbency, stupor, and sometimes convulsion. Hypocalcemia alone is infrequently recognized; laboratory data reflecting a primary disease commonly include hypocalcemia.

INTERPRETATION OF LABORATORY DATA

Decreased serum calcium concentration is sometimes accompanied by hypomagnesemia, hypermagnesemia, hypophosphatemia, or hyperphosphatemia. Decreased albumin concentration will lower total calcium concentration while ionized calcium concentration remains normal. Therefore, the total calcium concentration must be evaluated with the albumin concentration, or ionized calcium should be measured.

SIGNIFICANT DISEASES TO RULE OUT

- ◆ Tetanus often occurs following a wound. There is a normal serum calcium concentration.
- ◆ Exertional rhabdomyolysis causes severe muscle pain and markedly increased serum concentrations of CK and AST.

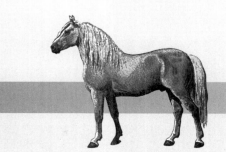

Signs

- ◆ Increased muscle tone
- ◆ Stiffness
- ◆ Trismus
- ◆ Sweating
- ◆ Muscle fasciculations
- ◆ Recumbency
- ◆ Stupor
- ◆ Convulsion

Serum Chemistry

	low	normal	high
CK			
AST			
SDH			
GGT			
bile acids			
bilirubin, total			
bilirubin, direct			
protein, total			
albumin			
globulin			
SUN			
creatinine			
glucose			
Ca	●		
P	●	●	●
Na			
K			
Cl			
tCO$_2$			

Hemogram

	low	normal	high
total RBC			
PCV			
total WBC			
neutrophils			
bands			
lymphocytes			
monocytes			
eosinophils			
basophils			
platelets			
fibrinogen			

Urinalysis

	normal	abnormal
color		
blood		
protein		
albumin		
glucose		
pH		
specific gravity		
WBC		
RBC		
epithelial cells		
bacteria		
casts		
crystals		

Special Tests

- ◆ Ionized calcium concentration is decreased.
- ◆ Hypomagnesemia or hypermagnesemia could accompany hypocalcemia.

- ● Changes caused by the disease itself
- ●† Changes secondary to dysfunction caused by the disease

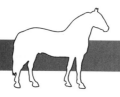

Reproductive System Diseases

Uterine infection

Granulosa-theca cell tumors

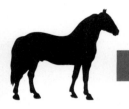

UTERINE INFECTION

Bacterial endometritis is uterine infection involving the endometrium and resulting in infertility and abnormalities in the interestrus interval. A purulent vaginal discharge is sometimes present. Septic metritis is inflammation of all layers of the uterine wall that develops within a few days after parturition. Clinical signs of septic metritis are fever, depression, anorexia, and laminitis. Vaginal discharge varies from scant white mucus to profuse malodorous red-black fluid. Metritis may or may not be associated with retained placenta. Vaginitis and cervicitis frequently accompany endometritis or metritis.

INTERPRETATION OF LABORATORY DATA

Mares with septic metritis usually develop neutropenia and leukopenia as a result of endotoxemia. Mares with chronic bacterial endometritis sometimes have total leukocyte counts below the normal range and mild nonregenerative anemia.

SIGNIFICANT DISEASES TO RULE OUT

◆ Vaginitis/cervicitis can be differentiated by results of vaginal and rectal examination.

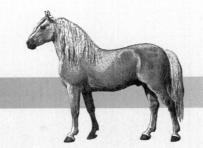

Signs

- ◆ Fever
- ◆ Depression
- ◆ Anorexia
- ◆ Laminitis
- ◆ Vaginal discharge

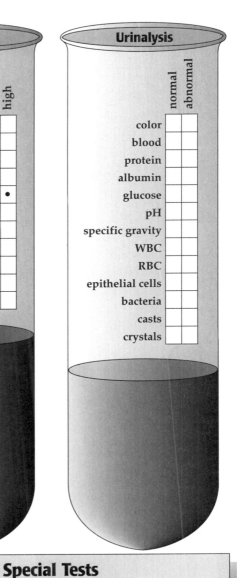

Serum Chemistry

	low	normal	high
CK			
AST			
SDH			
GGT			
bile acids			
bilirubin, total			
bilirubin, direct			
protein, total			
albumin			
globulin			
SUN			
creatinine			
glucose			
Ca			
P			
Na			
K			
Cl			
tCO$_2$			

Hemogram

	low	normal	high
total RBC	•	•	
PCV	•	•	
total WBC	•	•	
neutrophils	•	•	
bands		•	•
lymphocytes			
monocytes			
eosinophils			
basophils			
platelets			
fibrinogen			

Urinalysis

	normal	abnormal
color		
blood		
protein		
albumin		
glucose		
pH		
specific gravity		
WBC		
RBC		
epithelial cells		
bacteria		
casts		
crystals		

Special Tests

- ◆ Uterine culture may reveal the causative organism.

- • Changes caused by the disease itself
- •† Changes secondary to dysfunction caused by the disease

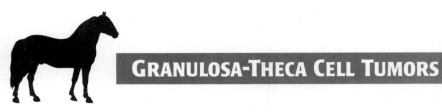

GRANULOSA-THECA CELL TUMORS

These are usually benign unilateral tumors of the ovary. Affected mares display either no clinical signs, anestrus, constant or intermittent estrus, or stallion-like behavior. Some mares show signs of abdominal discomfort. Palpation of the ovaries reveals multicystic enlargement of one ovary and atrophy of the contralateral ovary.

INTERPRETATION OF LABORATORY DATA

Concentrations of testosterone in the peripheral blood are usually increased above 50 pg/ml. Normal testosterone concentration in nonpregnant mares is less than 50 pg/ml, while elevations above 50 pg/ml may occur in normal pregnant mares.

SIGNIFICANT DISEASES TO RULE OUT

◆ Ovarian hematoma and abscess are differentiated by determining that the contralateral ovary and plasma testosterone concentrations are normal.

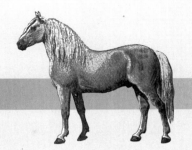

Signs

◆ No signs
◆ Anestrus
◆ Abnormal estrus
◆ Stallion-like
   behavior

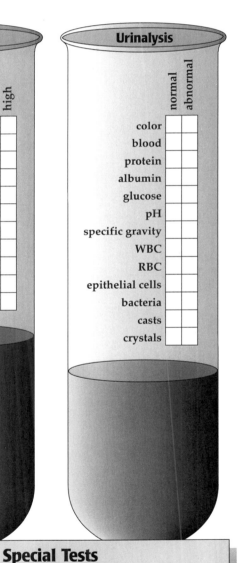

Serum Chemistry

	low	normal	high
CK			
AST			
SDH			
GGT			
bile acids			
bilirubin, total			
bilirubin, direct			
protein, total			
albumin			
globulin			
SUN			
creatinine			
glucose			
Ca			
P			
Na			
K			
Cl			
tCO$_2$			

Hemogram

	low	normal	high
total RBC			
PCV			
total WBC			
neutrophils			
bands			
lymphocytes			
monocytes			
eosinophils			
basophils			
platelets			
fibrinogen			

Urinalysis

	normal	abnormal
color		
blood		
protein		
albumin		
glucose		
pH		
specific gravity		
WBC		
RBC		
epithelial cells		
bacteria		
casts		
crystals		

Special Tests

◆ Concentrations of testosterone in the peripheral
   blood are increased.

● Changes caused by the disease itself
●† Changes secondary to dysfunction
   caused by the disease

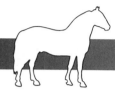

Endocrine System Diseases

Pituitary adenoma (equine Cushing's disease)

Adrenal insufficiency

Hypothyroidism

Nutritional secondary hyperparathyroidism

Diabetes mellitus

Abnormalities of ADH

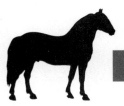

PITUITARY ADENOMA (EQUINE CUSHING'S DISEASE)

Functional adenomas or adenomatous hyperplasia of the pituitary pars intermedia can lead to hirsutism, recurrent laminitis and sole abscesses, polyuria, polydipsia, and hyperhidrosis. Clinical signs can result from excess circulating glucocorticoids, physical destruction of the pars nervosa, and increased circulating concentrations of other pituitary-derived peptides.

INTERPRETATION OF LABORATORY DATA

Horses with pituitary adenoma frequently have a normal CBC and chemistry panel. However, increased neutrophil counts and decreased lymphocyte counts are common because of hypercortisolemia. Concurrent infection may cause neutrophilia, hyperfibrinogenemia, and nonregenerative anemia. Hyperglycemia and glucosuria are present in many cases. Ketonemia sometimes occurs, causing ketonuria. Physical destruction of the pars nervosa by the enlarged pars media may decrease ADH secretion, resulting in urine dilution. Liver enzymes may be increased as a result of the effects of hypercortisolemia.

SIGNIFICANT DISEASES TO RULE OUT

- ◆ Renal disease will cause dilute urine and azotemia.
- ◆ Pheochromocytoma is characterized clinically by tachycardia, anxiety, hyperhidrosis, and dilated pupils.

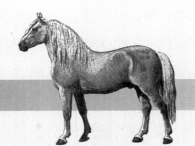

Signs

- ◆ Hirsutism
- ◆ Recurrent laminitis and sole abscesses
- ◆ Hyperhidrosis

Serum Chemistry

	low	normal	high
CK			
AST		•	•
SDH		•	•
GGT		•	•
bile acids			
bilirubin, total			
bilirubin, direct			
protein, total			
albumin			
globulin			
SUN			
creatinine			
glucose		•	•
Ca			
P			
Na			
K			
Cl			
tCO$_2$			

Hemogram

	low	normal	high
total RBC	•	•	
PCV	•	•	
total WBC		•	•
neutrophils		•	•
bands			
lymphocytes	•	•	
monocytes			
eosinophils			
basophils			
platelets			
fibrinogen		•	•

Urinalysis

	normal	abnormal
color		
blood		
protein		
albumin		
glucose	•	•
pH		
specific gravity	•	•
WBC		
RBC		
epithelial cells		
bacteria		
casts		
crystals		

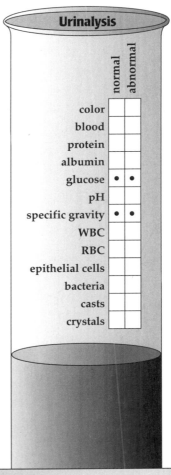

Special Tests

- ◆ Plasma cortisol concentration infrequently is increased.
- ◆ Dexamethasone administration partially or transiently suppresses plasma cortisol concentration.
- ◆ TRH administration increases plasma cortisol.
- ◆ Ketonuria rarely is detected on urine dipstick.

- • Changes caused by the disease itself
- •† Changes secondary to dysfunction caused by the disease

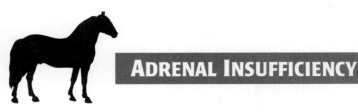

ADRENAL INSUFFICIENCY

Poor performance in race horses and endurance horses rarely has been attributed to adrenal insufficiency. These horses often show depression and anorexia. Frequently, the historical findings include intensive exercise performance, corticosteroid administration, or severe disease.

INTERPRETATION OF LABORATORY DATA

Although very little is known about this syndrome in horses, hyponatremia, hypochloremia, hyperkalemia, and hypoglycemia could result from glucocorticoid or mineralocorticoid deficiency. Low plasma cortisol concentrations are not always found in horses suspected to have this condition.

SIGNIFICANT DISEASES TO RULE OUT

◆ Renal failure will increase creatinine and SUN concentrations.
◆ Chronic liver failure will increase serum bilirubin, AST, SDH, and GGT activities.

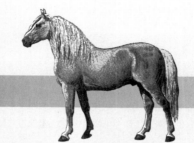

Signs

- ◆ Poor performance
- ◆ Anorexia
- ◆ Depression

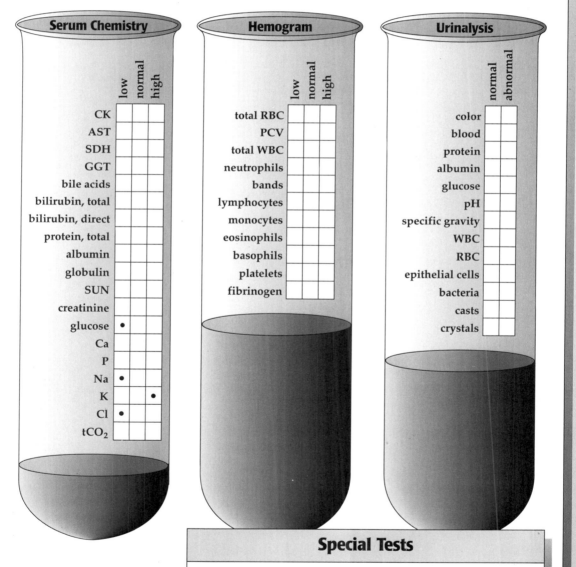

Serum Chemistry

	low	normal	high
CK			
AST			
SDH			
GGT			
bile acids			
bilirubin, total			
bilirubin, direct			
protein, total			
albumin			
globulin			
SUN			
creatinine			
glucose	•		
Ca			
P			
Na	•		
K			•
Cl	•		
tCO₂			

Hemogram

	low	normal	high
total RBC			
PCV			
total WBC			
neutrophils			
bands			
lymphocytes			
monocytes			
eosinophils			
basophils			
platelets			
fibrinogen			

Urinalysis

	normal	abnormal
color		
blood		
protein		
albumin		
glucose		
pH		
specific gravity		
WBC		
RBC		
epithelial cells		
bacteria		
casts		
crystals		

Special Tests

- ◆ Plasma cortisol concentration may be decreased.
- ◆ Response to ACTH stimulation is decreased.

- • Changes caused by the disease itself
- •† Changes secondary to dysfunction caused by the disease

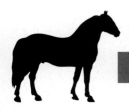

HYPOTHYROIDISM

Although hypothyroidism has not been documented in adult horses, it may rarely occur. Response to thyroid replacement has been documented in adult horses with scaly hair coat and decreased exercise performance. Hypothermia, edema, and decreased appetite have also been reported. Neonatal hypothyroidism has been documented in foals born to mares ingesting excessive quantities of iodine during pregnancy. Clinical signs in foals include goiter, incoordination, poor sucking and righting reflexes, hypothermia, tendon contracture or rupture, and tarsal collapse.

INTERPRETATION OF LABORATORY DATA

Baseline T_3 and T_4 concentrations are extremely variable; however, decreased concentrations have been obtained in horses with compatible clinical signs. Thyroid-stimulating hormone test provides a more reliable method of diagnosis.

SIGNIFICANT DISEASES TO RULE OUT

◆ Many other diseases can cause these vague clinical signs and decrease baseline thyroid hormone concentrations. Diagnosis is based on ruling out other conditions, performing TSH test, and monitoring response to therapy.

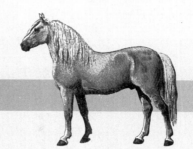

Signs

- ◆ Poor hair coat
- ◆ Poor performance
- ◆ Edema
- ◆ Anorexia

Serum Chemistry

	low	normal	high
CK			
AST			
SDH			
GGT			
bile acids			
bilirubin, total			
bilirubin, direct			
protein, total			
albumin			
globulin			
SUN			
creatinine			
glucose			
Ca			
P			
Na			
K			
Cl			
tCO$_2$			

Hemogram

	low	normal	high
total RBC			
PCV			
total WBC			
neutrophils			
bands			
lymphocytes			
monocytes			
eosinophils			
basophils			
platelets			
fibrinogen			

Urinalysis

	normal	abnormal
color		
blood		
protein		
albumin		
glucose		
pH		
specific gravity		
WBC		
RBC		
epithelial cells		
bacteria		
casts		
crystals		

Special Tests

- ◆ Serum concentration of thyroid hormones is decreased.
- ◆ The response to TSH administration is decreased.

• Changes caused by the disease itself

•† Changes secondary to dysfunction caused by the disease

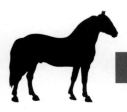

NUTRITIONAL SECONDARY HYPERPARATHYROIDISM

Nutritional secondary hyperparathyroidism occurs when horses ingest diets that are low in calcium and/or high in phosphorus. In an effort to maintain homeostasis, parathyroid hormone is released to mobilize calcium from bone and increase renal resorption of calcium and excretion of phosphorus. Clinical signs include shifting lameness and a stiff stilted gait. Facial bone distortion results in broadening of the face and thickening of the rami of the mandible.

INTERPRETATION OF LABORATORY DATA

Serum calcium concentration is normal. Serum phosphorus concentration is normal or slightly increased. Diagnosis is made by demonstration of increased renal fractional excretion of phosphorus with other compatible clinical findings.

DISEASES TO RULE OUT

◆ Laminitis can occur as a primary problem or secondary to nutritional secondary hyperparathyroidism.
◆ Facial bone distortion can result from neoplasia (osteoma, fibrosarcoma, squamous cell carcinoma). Radiography and bone biopsy help differentiate neoplasia from nutritional secondary hyperparathyroidism.

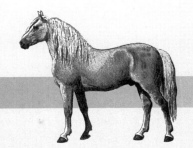

Signs

- ◆ Shifting leg lameness
- ◆ Stiff gait
- ◆ Facial bone distortion

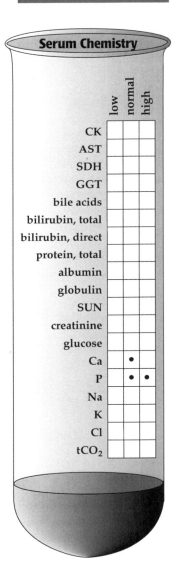

Serum Chemistry

	low	normal	high
CK			
AST			
SDH			
GGT			
bile acids			
bilirubin, total			
bilirubin, direct			
protein, total			
albumin			
globulin			
SUN			
creatinine			
glucose			
Ca		•	
P		•	•
Na			
K			
Cl			
tCO$_2$			

Hemogram

	low	normal	high
total RBC			
PCV			
total WBC			
neutrophils			
bands			
lymphocytes			
monocytes			
eosinophils			
basophils			
platelets			
fibrinogen			

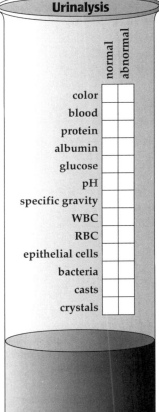

Urinalysis

	normal	abnormal
color		
blood		
protein		
albumin		
glucose		
pH		
specific gravity		
WBC		
RBC		
epithelial cells		
bacteria		
casts		
crystals		

Special Tests

- ◆ Renal fractional excretion of phosphorus is increased.
- ◆ Radiography reveals generalized loss of bone density and loss of cortical bone.
- ◆ Histology of bone biopsy reveals fibrous osteodystrophy.
- ◆ Analysis of mineral content of diet reveals decreased Ca:P ratio.

- • Changes caused by the disease itself
- •† Changes secondary to dysfunction caused by the disease

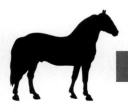

DIABETES MELLITUS

Diabetes mellitus results from hypoinsulinemia, excess concentration of counterregulatory hormones (e.g., cortisol), or tissue insensitivity to insulin. The most common form of diabetes mellitus in horses is secondary diabetes resulting from excess production of cortisol due to pituitary adenoma. Acquired non-insulin-dependent diabetes mellitus has been reported in obese ponies. The insensitivity of tissues to insulin and hyperinsulinemia in the ponies is associated with body condition. Weight loss from dietary control will return insulin concentrations to normal. Clinical signs include those associated with the primary problem (pituitary adenoma or obesity in ponies) and polyuria and polydipsia.

INTERPRETATION OF LABORATORY DATA

Horses with diabetes mellitus associated with pituitary adenoma may have increased neutrophil counts and decreased lymphocyte counts. Hyperglycemia and glucosuria are common. Ketonemia sometimes causes ketonuria. Liver enzymes may be increased as a result of the effects of hypercortisolemia.

Obese ponies may demonstrate hyperglycemia, glucosuria, and hyperinsulinemia.

DISEASES TO RULE OUT

◆ Pituitary adenoma is diagnosed by typical clinical signs and abnormal dexamethasone suppression test results.
◆ Central diabetes insipidus is caused by pituitary adenoma or is idiopathic.

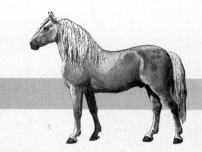

Signs

- ◆ Polyuria and polydipsia
- ◆ Obesity or hirsutism
- ◆ Hyperhidrosis
- ◆ Laminitis

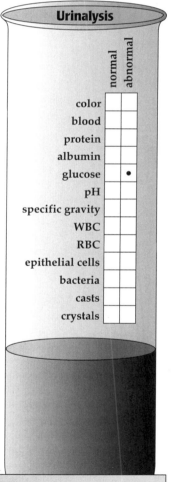

Serum Chemistry

	low	normal	high
CK			
AST		•	•
SDH		•	•
GGT		•	•
bile acids			
bilirubin, total			
bilirubin, direct			
protein, total			
albumin			
globulin			
SUN			
creatinine			
glucose			•
Ca			
P			
Na			
K			
Cl			
tCO$_2$			

Hemogram

	low	normal	high
total RBC			
PCV			
total WBC			
neutrophils		•	•
bands			
lymphocytes	•	•	
monocytes			
eosinophils			
basophils			
platelets			
fibrinogen			

Urinalysis

	normal	abnormal
color		
blood		
protein		
albumin		
glucose		•
pH		
specific gravity		
WBC		
RBC		
epithelial cells		
bacteria		
casts		
crystals		

Special Tests

- ◆ Dexamethasone suppression and TRH stimulation tests are abnormal in horses with diabetes secondary to pituitary adenoma.
- ◆ Obese ponies have hyperinsulinemia.
- ◆ Urine dipstick may be positive for ketones.

• Changes caused by the disease itself

•† Changes secondary to dysfunction caused by the disease

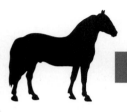

ABNORMALITIES OF ANTIDIURETIC HORMONE (ADH)

Decreased production of ADH results from diseases of the hypothalamus. Pituitary adenoma is the most common disease, but idiopathic central diabetes insipidus has been reported in a horse. Polyuria and polydipsia are the predominant clinical signs.

Increased production of ADH (inappropriate ADH) has not been documented in horses. Suspected cases have resulted from severe shock due to endotoxemia associated with gastrointestinal disease. Peripheral edema and decreased urine production may be caused by excessive production of ADH.

INTERPRETATION OF LABORATORY DATA

Decreased production of ADH will result in urine dilution (specific gravity less than 1.008). Pituitary adenoma may be accompanied by neutrophilia, lymphopenia, hyperglycemia, glucosuria, and increased liver enzymes.

Increased production of ADH causes hyponatremia and concentrated urine.

SIGNIFICANT DISEASES TO RULE OUT

- Pituitary adenoma is the most common cause of decreased ADH production and is diagnosed by dexamethasone suppression testing.
- Chronic renal failure causes polyuria, isosthenuria, proteinuria, and azotemia.
- Acute renal failure can cause oliguria, peripheral edema, and hyponatremia. There is severe azotemia and isosthenuria with acute renal failure.

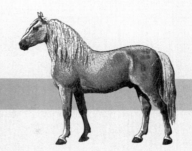

Signs

◆ Polyuria and polydipsia

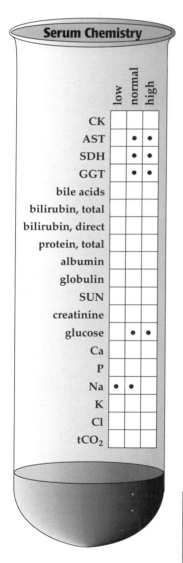

Serum Chemistry

	low	normal	high
CK			
AST		•	•
SDH		•	•
GGT		•	•
bile acids			
bilirubin, total			
bilirubin, direct			
protein, total			
albumin			
globulin			
SUN			
creatinine			
glucose		•	•
Ca			
P			
Na	•	•	
K			
Cl			
tCO$_2$			

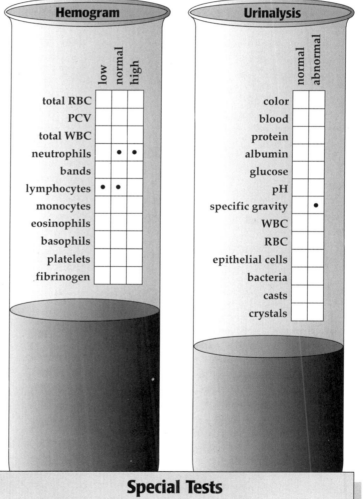

Hemogram

	low	normal	high
total RBC			
PCV			
total WBC			
neutrophils		•	•
bands			
lymphocytes	•	•	
monocytes			
eosinophils			
basophils			
platelets			
fibrinogen			

Urinalysis

	normal	abnormal
color		
blood		
protein		
albumin		
glucose		
pH		
specific gravity		•
WBC		
RBC		
epithelial cells		
bacteria		
casts		
crystals		

Special Tests

◆ Horses with decreased production of ADH from pituitary adenoma will have abnormal dexamethasone suppression testing.
◆ ADH administration will result in urine concentration.

• Changes caused by the disease itself
•† Changes secondary to dysfunction caused by the disease

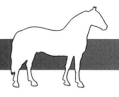

Hematologic Diseases

Acute blood loss

Chronic blood loss

Hemolytic anemia

Immune-mediated thrombocytopenia

Disseminated intravascular coagulation

Warfarin toxicosis

Plasma-cell myeloma

Malignant lymphoma

Neonatal isoerythrolysis

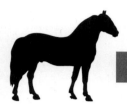

Acute Blood Loss

Initial acute blood loss may present with a normal PCV resulting from splenic contraction. Restoration of the blood volume begins about 3 hours following the hemorrhage, so that by 72 hours the erythrocyte mass is diluted and laboratory signs of anemia are evident. Acute blood loss may be caused by trauma, surgery, gastrointestinal ulcers, or hemostasis defects. Clinical signs are depression, weakness, tachycardia, tachypnea, pale mucous membranes, and possibly hypovolemic shock.

Interpretation of Laboratory Data

The PCV and plasma protein are decreased. During the first hours following acute blood loss, platelet numbers may be increased and a neutrophilic leukocytosis occurs. Reticulocytes, or polychromatophilic cells, are not released into the peripheral blood of horses even in the presence of a regenerative anemia, but anisocytosis due to a macrocytosis may be evident with a maximal response. By 48 to 72 hours erythroid hyperplasia and reticulocytosis are evident in the bone marrow. Hepatic hypoxia may produce increased serum SDH and AST activities; metabolic acidosis (decreased tCO_2) may occur.

Significant Diseases to Rule Out

◆ Chronic blood loss can be ruled out by the history and by bone marrow evaluation. Marrow evaluation of anemia of chronic blood loss will reveal decreased iron stores and lack of erythrocyte regeneration.
◆ Cardiac disease will usually have signs of murmur or arrhythmia.
◆ Respiratory disease will present with abnormal findings on respiratory examination.

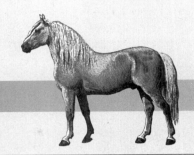

Signs

◆ Depression
◆ Weakness
◆ Tachycardia
◆ Tachypnea
◆ Pale mucous membranes
◆ Hypovolemic shock

Serum Chemistry

	low	normal	high
CK			
AST		•	•†
SDH		•	•†
GGT			
bile acids			
bilirubin, total			
bilirubin, direct			
protein, total	•	•	
albumin	•	•	
globulin	•	•	
SUN			
creatinine			
glucose			
Ca			
P			
Na			
K			
Cl			
tCO₂	•	•	

Hemogram

	low	normal	high
total RBC	•	•	
PCV	•	•	
total WBC		•	•
neutrophils		•	•
bands			
lymphocytes			
monocytes			
eosinophils			
basophils			
platelets		•	•
fibrinogen			

Urinalysis

	normal	abnormal
color		
blood		
protein		
albumin		
glucose		
pH		
specific gravity		
WBC		
RBC		
epithelial cells		
bacteria		
casts		
crystals		

Special Tests

◆ Bone marrow will show erythroid hyperplasia.

• Changes caused by the disease itself

•† Changes secondary to dysfunction caused by the disease

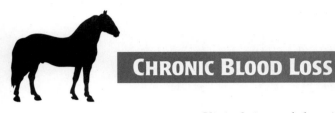

CHRONIC BLOOD LOSS

Clinical signs of chronic blood loss can include depression, weakness, pale mucous membranes, exercise intolerance, and a systolic murmur. However, these signs may be masked because the anemia develops slowly, giving the animal time to adapt. Chronic blood loss may be the result of parasitism, thrombocytopenia, gastrointestinal ulcers, hematuria, or neoplasia. Chronic blood loss anemia is usually more severe with external blood loss and may progress to nonregenerative iron-lack anemia. Internal blood loss is usually less severe and somewhat regenerative.

INTERPRETATION OF LABORATORY DATA

The PCV is decreased and hypoproteinemia is usually observed. Thrombocytosis can be seen. Erythrocyte poikilocytosis, low serum iron, increased total iron-binding capacity, and absence of bone marrow macrophage iron indicate that an external blood loss has progressed to iron-lack anemia. Increased serum SDH and AST activities may result from hepatic hypoxia.

SIGNIFICANT DISEASES TO RULE OUT

◆ Cardiac disease will usually have signs of murmur or arrhythmia.
◆ Respiratory disease will present with abnormal findings on respiratory examination.

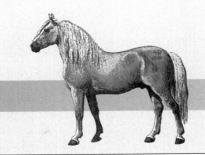

Signs

◆ Depression
◆ Weakness
◆ Pale mucous
  membranes
◆ Exercise
  intolerance
◆ Systolic murmur

Serum Chemistry

	low	normal	high
CK			
AST		•	•†
SDH		•	•†
GGT			
bile acids			
bilirubin, total			
bilirubin, direct			
protein, total	•		
albumin	•		
globulin	•		
SUN			
creatinine			
glucose			
Ca			
P			
Na			
K			
Cl			
tCO₂			

Hemogram

	low	normal	high
total RBC	•		
PCV	•		
total WBC			
neutrophils			
bands			
lymphocytes			
monocytes			
eosinophils			
basophils			
platelets		•	•
fibrinogen			

Urinalysis

	normal	abnormal
color		
blood		
protein		
albumin		
glucose		
pH		
specific gravity		
WBC		
RBC		
epithelial cells		
bacteria		
casts		
crystals		

Special Tests

◆ Bone marrow aspiration may reveal lack of iron
  stores.
◆ Fecal testing for occult blood may be positive.
◆ Serum iron will be decreased and TIBC levels will
  be increased.

• Changes caused by the disease itself
•† Changes secondary to dysfunction
   caused by the disease

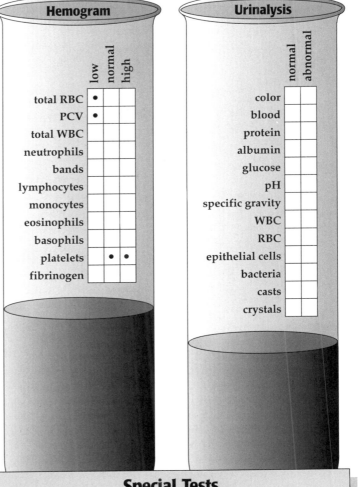

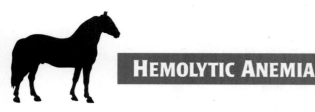

HEMOLYTIC ANEMIA

Hemolytic anemia may be caused by infectious diseases (EIA, babesiosis), immune-mediated mechanisms, or erythrocyte oxidative damage (red maple, onion, phenothiazine toxicosis). Hemolysis has been observed in terminal cases of liver failure. In cases of infectious or immune-mediated anemia (EIA, babesiosis), antibody attaches to the erythrocyte surface, resulting in complement-mediated lysis or phagocytosis and early removal from circulation. Red maple and onion toxicosis cause alteration in the structure of hemoglobin, resulting in Heinz body formation or eccentrocytes. Clinical signs include icterus, fever, weakness, depression, and hemoglobinuria.

INTERPRETATION OF LABORATORY DATA

Icterus, hemoglobinemia, and/or hemoglobinuria, and refractometric hyperproteinemia may occur with intravascular hemolytic anemias (babesiosis, red maple, liver failure, immune-mediated). Heinz bodies and eccentrocytes are erythrocyte changes specifically associated with oxidative hemolytic anemias (red maple). These cells are more easily identified with new methylene blue staining. A brown discoloration of serum resulting from methemoglobinemia may also occur. EIA usually presents with extravascular hemolysis and is often accompanied by neutropenia and thrombocytopenia. Monocyte phagocytosis of erythrocytes can result in the production of spherocytes. Coombs testing may detect the presence of antibody on the erythrocytes. Hemolytic anemias are normally characterized by a marked regenerative response. By 48 to 72 hours marked erythroid hyperplasia and reticulocytosis are evident in the bone marrow; however, horses with regenerative anemias do not exhibit polychromasia in the peripheral blood.

Hemoglobinuria, indicated by brownish-red coloration of the urine, can cause toxic damage to renal tubular epithelial cells, progressing to renal failure. Urinalysis will reveal casts and isosthenuria; serum creatinine and SUN concentrations are increased. Ammonium sulfate will precipitate hemoglobin from the urine. Animals may experience metabolic acidosis (decreased tCO_2). Increased serum SDH and AST activities may result from hepatic hypoxia.

SIGNIFICANT DISEASES TO RULE OUT

- Hyperbilirubinemia resulting from anorexia may exhibit a marked hyperbilirubinemia without anemia.
- Acute blood loss can be differentiated from extravascular hemolytic anemia by identifying sources of blood loss and decreased total protein.
- Hemolytic anemia of liver failure reveals increases in hepatocellular enzyme activities and abnormal liver function tests.

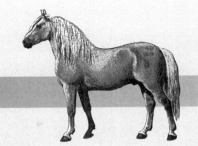

Signs

- ◆ Fever
- ◆ Depression
- ◆ Weakness
- ◆ Icterus
- ◆ Hemoglobinuria

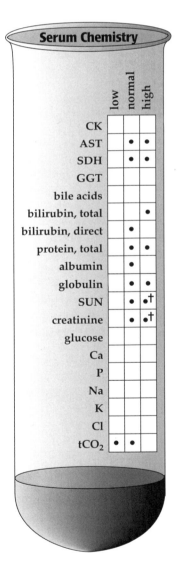

Serum Chemistry

	low	normal	high
CK			
AST		•	•
SDH		•	•
GGT			
bile acids			
bilirubin, total			•
bilirubin, direct		•	
protein, total		•	•
albumin		•	
globulin		•	•
SUN		•	•†
creatinine		•	•†
glucose			
Ca			
P			
Na			
K			
Cl			
tCO₂	•	•	

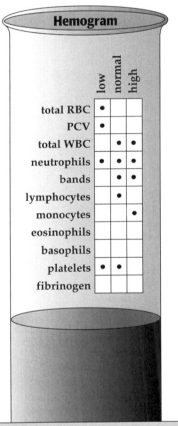

Hemogram

	low	normal	high
total RBC	•		
PCV	•		
total WBC		•	•
neutrophils	•	•	•
bands		•	•
lymphocytes		•	
monocytes			•
eosinophils			
basophils			
platelets	•	•	
fibrinogen			

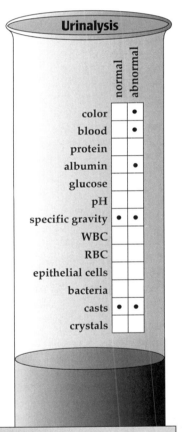

Urinalysis

	normal	abnormal
color		•
blood		•
protein		
albumin		•
glucose		
pH		
specific gravity	•	•
WBC		
RBC		
epithelial cells		
bacteria		
casts	•	•
crystals		

Special Tests

- ◆ Blood smear may reveal presence of Heinz bodies, eccentrocytes, spherocytes, erythroparasites.
- ◆ Coggins' test may be positive.
- ◆ Bone marrow aspirate will indicate a regenerative response.
- ◆ Coombs' test may be positive.
- ◆ Hemoglobinuria can be differentiated from myoglobinuria by presence of red plasma and precipitation after addition of ammonium sulfate to urine.

- • Changes caused by the disease itself
- •† Changes secondary to dysfunction caused by the disease

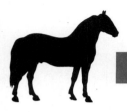

IMMUNE-MEDIATED THROMBOCYTOPENIA

Immune-mediated thrombocytopenia results from an increased destruction of platelets and/or a decreased production by megakaryocytes following the formation of antibody to an antigen associated with either of these blood components. Immune-mediated thrombocytopenia may be primary idiopathic (absence of defined cause) or secondary to other disease conditions or to drug administration. In primary immune-mediated thrombocytopenia, antibody to cell membrane antigen may coat either platelets or megakaryocytes, resulting in premature removal of the platelets or decreased production by megakaryocytes. In secondary immune-mediated thrombocytopenia, the immunoglobulin coating the platelets or megakaryocytes is directed against a specific drug, infectious agent, or neoplastic antigen bound to the membrane surface Fc receptor. Common clinical signs are mucosal petechiation, epistaxis, hyphema, and hemorrhagic tendencies from multiple sites.

INTERPRETATION OF LABORATORY DATA

In primary immune-mediated thrombocytopenia, a low platelet count ($< 40,000/\mu l$) is the principal laboratory finding. Other data include a prolonged bleeding time (> 5 min) and abnormal clot retraction. OSPT, APTT, and fibrinogen concentrations are normal. The ACT may be prolonged because of low platelet numbers. Urine and feces may be positive for occult blood, and if significant blood loss has occurred, anemia may be evident. Bone marrow evaluation usually reveals megakaryocytic hyperplasia, with or without large or shift platelets in the peripheral blood; however, if antibody is directed against megakaryocytes, bone marrow megakaryocytic hypoplasia is possible. Serum globulins concentration may be increased. Definitive diagnosis by demonstration of increased quantities of antiplatelet antibody or platelet-associated Ig, or by the platelet factor 3 immunoinjury assay, is not established in horses.

SIGNIFICANT DISEASES TO RULE OUT

◆ Vasculitis usually demonstrates a normal platelet count.
◆ Pseudothrombocytopenia is an artifactually low count due to EDTA-induced platelet clumping. Collecting blood for the platelet count in 3.8% sodium citrate will eliminate this problem.
◆ Spuriously low counts can occur as a result of improper blood collection and handling. Count will be normal with a proper venipuncture.
◆ Myelophthisic diseases can be determined by bone marrow aspiration with observation of replacement by other cells.
◆ Disseminated intravascular coagulation occurs secondary to a primary disease process. OSPT and APTT are prolonged.

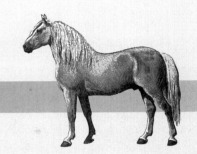

Signs

- Mucosal petechiae
- Epistaxis
- Melena
- Hyphema
- Hemorrhagic tendencies from multiple sites

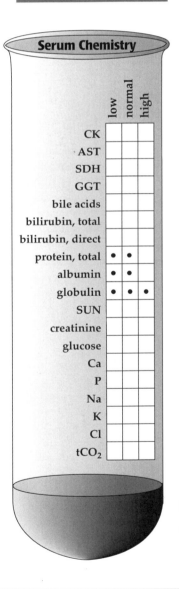

Serum Chemistry

	low	normal	high
CK			
AST			
SDH			
GGT			
bile acids			
bilirubin, total			
bilirubin, direct			
protein, total	•	•	
albumin	•	•	
globulin	•	•	•
SUN			
creatinine			
glucose			
Ca			
P			
Na			
K			
Cl			
tCO$_2$			

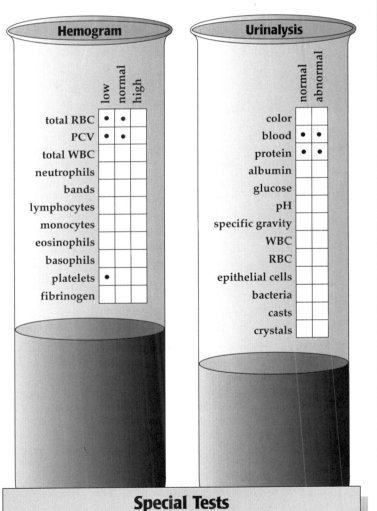

Hemogram

	low	normal	high
total RBC	•	•	
PCV	•	•	
total WBC			
neutrophils			
bands			
lymphocytes			
monocytes			
eosinophils			
basophils			
platelets	•		
fibrinogen			

Urinalysis

	normal	abnormal
color		
blood	•	•
protein	•	•
albumin		
glucose		
pH		
specific gravity		
WBC		
RBC		
epithelial cells		
bacteria		
casts		
crystals		

Special Tests

- Bleeding time will be prolonged.
- Fecal occult blood may be positive.
- Bone marrow evaluation may reveal abnormal megakaryocyte numbers or maturation.
- ACT may be prolonged.

• Changes caused by the disease itself

•† Changes secondary to dysfunction caused by the disease

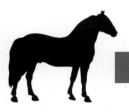

DISSEMINATED INTRAVASCULAR COAGULATION

Disseminated intravascular coagulation (DIC) may occur with gastro-intestinal disorders, laminitis, neoplasia, endotoxemia, septicemia, necrosis, intravascular hemolysis, heat stroke, shock, dehydration, polycythemia, and other conditions. Many body systems can be involved. Excessive thrombin formation occurs and coagulation factors and platelets are depleted. In addition to fever, hemorrhagic tendencies from multiple sites, and rapidly progressive shock, clinical signs are related to the predisposing disease.

INTERPRETATION OF LABORATORY DATA

Platelet numbers are usually less than 90,000/μl; OSPT and APTT are prolonged; fibrin/fibrinogen degradation products (FDP) are increased. Plasma fibrinogen concentration can be increased early in the process. With chronic DIC, findings may be within normal limits, except for an increased concentration of FDP. Other laboratory data may reflect the primary disease process or resulting organ failure (increased AST, SDH, and GGT activities, increased bilirubin and bile acid concentrations, decreased glucose, and increased creatinine and SUN concentrations).

SIGNIFICANT DISEASES TO RULE OUT

- ◆ (A primary disease process will always be present prior to DIC.)
- ◆ Immune-mediated thrombocytopenia does not cause prolongation of OSPT and APTT tests.
- ◆ Coagulation factor defects do not result in decreased platelet numbers.

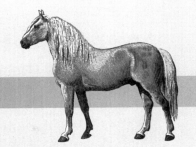

Signs

- ◆ Fever
- ◆ Hemorrhagic tendencies
- ◆ Rapidly progressive shock

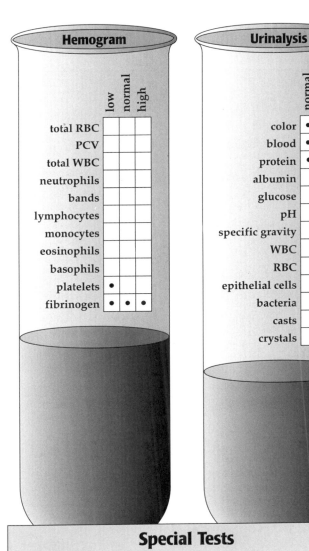

Serum Chemistry

	low	normal	high
CK			
AST		•	•†
SDH		•	•†
GGT		•	•†
bile acids		•	•†
bilirubin, total		•	•†
bilirubin, direct		•	•†
protein, total			
albumin			
globulin			
SUN			•†
creatinine			•†
glucose	•	•	
Ca			
P			
Na			
K			
Cl			
tCO₂			

Hemogram

	low	normal	high
total RBC			
PCV			
total WBC			
neutrophils			
bands			
lymphocytes			
monocytes			
eosinophils			
basophils			
platelets	•		
fibrinogen	•	•	•

Urinalysis

	normal	abnormal
color	•	•
blood	•	•
protein	•	•
albumin		
glucose		
pH		
specific gravity		
WBC		
RBC		
epithelial cells		
bacteria		
casts		
crystals		

Special Tests

- ◆ ACT, APTT, OSPT, TCT are usually prolonged.
- ◆ FDP are increased.
- ◆ Fecal occult blood may be positive.

- • Changes caused by the disease itself
- •† Changes secondary to dysfunction caused by the disease

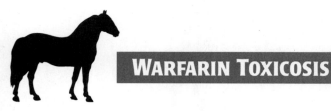

WARFARIN TOXICOSIS

Warfarin toxicosis is uncommon in horses. Moldy sweet clover, warfarin, and related compounds inhibit carboxylation and hence activity of vitamin K–dependent coagulation factors II, VII, IX, and X. Horses exhibit epistaxis, subcutaneous hematomas, hemorrhagic tendencies from multiple sites, and melena.

INTERPRETATION OF LABORATORY DATA

Laboratory data are consistent with multiple clotting factor deficiencies, so that both OSPT and APTT are prolonged. Because factor VII has the shortest half-life of the affected factors, a prolongation of OSPT occurs first. Plasma fibrinogen, platelet numbers, and fibrin/fibrinogen degradation products are normal. Fecal blood loss and hematuria may result in loss of total protein, albumin, and red blood cells.

SIGNIFICANT DISEASES TO RULE OUT

- Thrombocytopenia is diagnosed by a markedly decreased platelet count.
- DIC is diagnosed by a markedly decreased platelet count, increased concentrations of FDP, and an abnormally increased or decreased fibrinogen concentration.

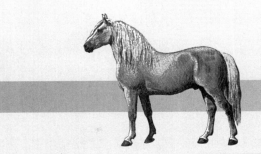

Signs

- Epistaxis
- Subcutaneous hematomas
- Melena
- Hemorrhagic tendencies

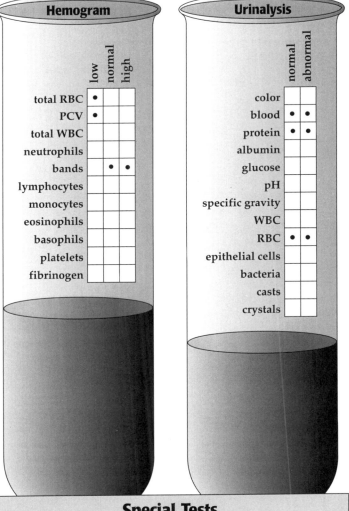

Serum Chemistry

	low	normal	high
CK			
AST			
SDH			
GGT			
bile acids			
bilirubin, total			
bilirubin, direct			
protein, total	•	•	
albumin	•	•	
globulin	•	•	
SUN			
creatinine			
glucose			
Ca			
P			
Na			
K			
Cl			
tCO$_2$			

Hemogram

	low	normal	high
total RBC	•		
PCV	•		
total WBC			
neutrophils			
bands		•	•
lymphocytes			
monocytes			
eosinophils			
basophils			
platelets			
fibrinogen			

Urinalysis

	normal	abnormal
color		
blood	•	•
protein	•	•
albumin		
glucose		
pH		
specific gravity		
WBC		
RBC	•	•
epithelial cells		
bacteria		
casts		
crystals		

Special Tests

- OSPT will become prolonged first, followed by prolongation of APTT.
- Fecal occult blood may be positive.

- Changes caused by the disease itself
- † Changes secondary to dysfunction caused by the disease

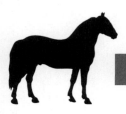

PLASMA-CELL MYELOMA

Plasma-cell myeloma is a very rare disease in horses. It is characterized by neoplastic proliferation of plasma cells in the bone marrow. Neoplastic cells sometimes invade the kidney, spleen, liver, and lymph nodes. Clinical signs include intermittent fever, weight loss, weakness, edema, hemorrhagic diathesis, and lameness. Renal failure and infections occasionally develop. Osteolysis is not a consistent finding in horses.

INTERPRETATION OF LABORATORY DATA

Diagnostic features of plasma-cell myeloma include a monoclonal gammopathy, >20% plasma cells in the bone marrow, radiographic evidence of osteolysis, and Bence Jones proteinuria. Horses become anemic and sometimes thrombocytopenic as the neoplastic cells crowd out normal bone marrow production. Hyperproteinemia is due to a monoclonal gammopathy. Animals are frequently azotemic as a result of renal involvement, and hyperviscosity syndrome and hypercalcemia can develop.

SIGNIFICANT DISEASES TO RULE OUT

◆ Other myeloproliferative disorders will not reveal neoplastic plasma cells in the bone marrow.
◆ Malignant lymphomas usually do not develop hyperviscosity syndrome, and neoplastic cells are not characteristic of plasma cells.

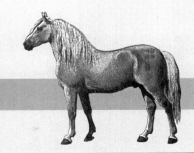

Signs

- ◆ Intermittent fever
- ◆ Weight loss
- ◆ Weakness
- ◆ Edema
- ◆ Hemorrhagic diathesis
- ◆ Lameness

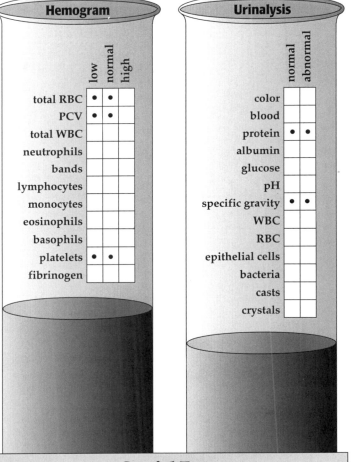

Serum Chemistry	low	normal	high
CK			
AST			
SDH			
GGT			
bile acids			
bilirubin, total			
bilirubin, direct			
protein, total			•
albumin	•	•	
globulin			•
SUN		•	•
creatinine		•	•
glucose			
Ca		•	•
P			
Na			
K			
Cl			
tCO₂			

Hemogram	low	normal	high
total RBC	•	•	
PCV	•	•	
total WBC			
neutrophils			
bands			
lymphocytes			
monocytes			
eosinophils			
basophils			
platelets	•	•	
fibrinogen			

Urinalysis	normal	abnormal
color		
blood		
protein	•	•
albumin		
glucose		
pH		
specific gravity	•	•
WBC		
RBC		
epithelial cells		
bacteria		
casts		
crystals		

Special Tests

- ◆ Protein electrophoresis reveals a monoclonal gammopathy.
- ◆ Radiographs may indicate osteolysis.
- ◆ Bence Jones proteins may be found in the urine.
- ◆ Bone marrow evaluation may reveal >20% plasma cells.

- • Changes caused by the disease itself
- •† Changes secondary to dysfunction caused by the disease

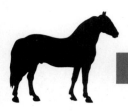

MALIGNANT LYMPHOMA

Malignant lymphoma affects all ages of horses, but is most common in adults. Malignant lymphoma may be manifested as a multicentric, alimentary, cutaneous, or mediastinal form. The disease is progressive, with animals exhibiting weight loss, diarrhea, depression, fever, lymphadenopathy, anorexia, venous distention, subcutaneous edema, and anemia. Other clinical signs represent the organ system involved.

INTERPRETATION OF LABORATORY DATA

Laboratory findings are variable, depending on locations and extent of tumor involvement. Horses may have nonregenerative anemia, neutrophilic leukocytosis, hyperglobulinemia, and hyperfibrinogenemia associated with chronic inflammatory disease. Protein electrophoresis may rarely detect a monoclonal gammopathy. Occasionally hypercalcemia occurs. Mediastinal or visceral involvement can result in thoracic or abdominal effusion containing neoplastic cells and increased protein. Hepatic involvement may induce increases in AST, SDH, and GGT activities. Hyperbilirubinemia can occur secondary to hepatic infiltration and anorexia. Anorexia may lead to hypokalemia. Gastrointestinal lymphosarcoma can cause malabsorption. Secondary immune-mediated anemia has been reported. Lymphocytic leukemia is unusual. Aspiration cytology or biopsy of tumor mass reveals a uniform population of neoplastic lymphocytes.

SIGNIFICANT DISEASES TO RULE OUT

◆ Plasma cell myeloma is differentiated by recognizing cellular morphology consistent with plasma cells, and finding neoplastic plasma cells in the bone marrow.
◆ Infiltrative intestinal disease other than lymphoma can be differentiated by biopsy.
◆ Hepatic diseases other than infiltrative lymphoma can be diagnosed by biopsy.

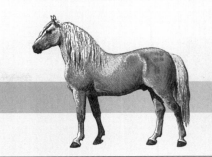

Signs

- ◆ Weight loss
- ◆ Diarrhea
- ◆ Depression
- ◆ Fever
- ◆ Lymph-
  adenopathy
- ◆ Anorexia
- ◆ Venous
  distention
- ◆ Subcutaneous
  edema
- ◆ Anemia

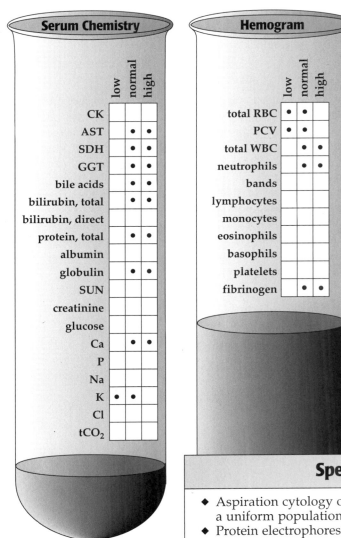

Serum Chemistry

	low	normal	high
CK			
AST		•	•
SDH		•	•
GGT		•	•
bile acids		•	•
bilirubin, total		•	•
bilirubin, direct			
protein, total		•	•
albumin			
globulin		•	•
SUN			
creatinine			
glucose			
Ca		•	•
P			
Na			
K	•	•	
Cl			
tCO₂			

Hemogram

	low	normal	high
total RBC	•	•	
PCV	•	•	
total WBC		•	•
neutrophils		•	•
bands			
lymphocytes			
monocytes			
eosinophils			
basophils			
platelets			
fibrinogen		•	•

Urinalysis

	normal	abnormal
color		
blood		
protein		
albumin		
glucose		
pH		
specific gravity		
WBC		
RBC		
epithelial cells		
bacteria		
casts		
crystals		

Special Tests

- ◆ Aspiration cytology or biopsy of tumor mass reveals a uniform population of neoplastic lymphocytes.
- ◆ Protein electrophoresis reveals polyclonal gammopathy or sometimes monoclonal gammopathy.
- ◆ Gastrointestinal lymphoma can cause xylose or glucose malabsorption.
- ◆ Coombs' test may be positive.

- • Changes caused by the disease itself
- •† Changes secondary to dysfunction caused by the disease

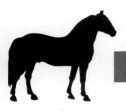

NEONATAL ISOERYTHROLYSIS

Neonatal isoerythrolysis is the destruction of red blood cells in the circulation of a foal by alloantibodies produced by the mare. These antibodies are excreted into colostrum and absorbed from the foal's intestinal tract in the first few hours of life. Foals are born healthy and begin to develop signs due to hemolysis and anemia at 24 to 36 hours after suckling. Clinical signs depend on the severity of the condition and include lethargy, weakness, reduced suckling, icteric mucous membranes, tachypnea, tachycardia, and hemoglobinuria.

INTERPRETATION OF LABORATORY DATA

All indicators of red blood cell concentration (packed cell volume, hemoglobin, and red blood cell count) are decreased. Serum bilirubin is markedly increased. Hemoglobinemia and hemoglobinuria may be detected on analysis of plasma and urine, respectively. Decreased fluid intake may cause dehydration, often resulting in prerenal azotemia. Hemoglobin is toxic to renal tubular cells, and, therefore, hemoglobinemia and hemoglobinuria may lead to renal azotemia. Renal failure will cause the urine specific gravity to be in the isosthenuric range (1.008 to 1.012). However, the urine specific gravity of foals normally is less than 1.010. Casts and blood may be seen in urine. Concurrent failure of passive transfer will lead to hypogammaglobulinemia. Decreased food intake may lead to hypoglycemia.

SIGNIFICANT DISEASES TO RULE OUT

◆ Septicemia does not cause anemia.
◆ Tyzzer's disease does not cause anemia, but causes elevation of serum liver enzyme activity.

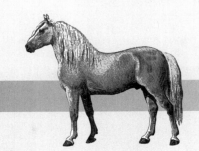

Signs

- ◆ Lethargy
- ◆ Weakness
- ◆ Reduced suckling
- ◆ Icterus
- ◆ Tachypnea
- ◆ Tachycardia
- ◆ Hemoglobinuria

Serum Chemistry

	low	normal	high
CK			
AST			
SDH			
GGT			
bile acids			
bilirubin, total		•	•
bilirubin, direct		•	•
protein, total			
albumin			
globulin			
SUN		•	
creatinine		•	
glucose	•†	•	
Ca			
P			
Na			
K			
Cl			
tCO₂			

Hemogram

	low	normal	high
total RBC	•		
PCV	•		
total WBC			
neutrophils			
bands			
lymphocytes			
monocytes			
eosinophils			
basophils			
platelets			
fibrinogen			

Urinalysis

	normal	abnormal
color	•	•
blood	•	•
protein	•	•
albumin		
glucose		
pH		
specific gravity	•	•
WBC	•	•
RBC	•	•
epithelial cells		
bacteria		
casts	•	•
crystals		

Special Tests

- ◆ Blood typing and cross matching (Serology Laboratory, University of California, Davis, CA) of mare and foal confirm the disease.
- ◆ Plasma may be discolored red.
- ◆ ELISA testing may reveal hypogammaglobulinemia.

• Changes caused by the disease itself

•† Changes secondary to dysfunction caused by the disease

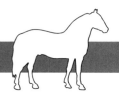

Immunologic Diseases

Failure of passive transfer

Combined immunodeficiency disease

IgM deficiency

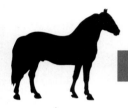

Failure of Passive Transfer

Failure of passive transfer of maternal immunoglobulin (FPT) is the most common immunologic disorder of foals. FPT may be complete or partial and may result from a failure of the foal to ingest an adequate volume of colostrum, from an inadequate concentration of Ig in the colostrum, or from lack of absorption of ingested colostrum. Clinical signs of sepsis are usually present within the first week of life.

Interpretation of Laboratory Data

Determination of plasma IgG concentrations should be performed on blood samples collected from the foal 18 to 24 hours after birth. Total serum protein or serum protein electrophoresis will provide estimates of immunoglobulin absorption; however, the ELISA test for quantitation of IgG is the most practical and accurate method for determination of immunoglobulin. Foals with IgG concentrations < 400 mg/dl at 24 hours are classified as having failure of passive transfer; foals with IgG concentrations >400 but <600 mg/dl are classified as having partial failure. Any concurrent perinatal conditions of the mare and foal should be considered in evaluating the foal's risk of sepsis. Laboratory changes consistent with sepsis can occur.

Significant Diseases to Rule Out

◆ Combined immunodeficiency reveals absence of serum IgM, lymphopenia (<1000/ml), and hypoplasia of lymphoid tissues.
◆ Other immunodeficient diseases are characterized clinically by persistent or recurrent infections. Diagnosis is made by low to absent concentrations of specific immunoglobulins and/or abnormal cell-mediated function. These diseases include:
   Agammaglobulinemia
   Selective IgM deficiency
   Transient hypogammaglobulinemia
   Partial immunodeficiency
   Partial cell-mediated immunodeficiency

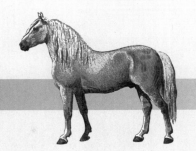

Signs

◆ Clinical signs are not present until condition progresses to sepsis

Serum Chemistry

	low	normal	high
CK			
AST			
SDH			
GGT			
bile acids			
bilirubin, total			
bilirubin, direct			
protein, total	●	●	
albumin		●	
globulin	●	●	
SUN			
creatinine			
glucose			
Ca			
P			
Na			
K			
Cl			
tCO$_2$			

Hemogram

	low	normal	high
total RBC			
PCV			
total WBC	●†	●	●†
neutrophils	●†	●	●†
bands		●	●†
lymphocytes			
monocytes			
eosinophils			
basophils			
platelets			
fibrinogen		●	●†

Urinalysis

	normal	abnormal
color		
blood		
protein		
albumin		
glucose		
pH		
specific gravity		
WBC		
RBC		
epithelial cells		
bacteria		
casts		
crystals		

Special Tests

◆ ELISA for level of plasma IgG will be <400 mg/dl at 24 hours.

● Changes caused by the disease itself

●† Changes secondary to dysfunction caused by the disease

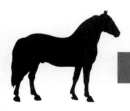

COMBINED IMMUNODEFICIENCY DISEASE (CID)

CID is a genetic and inherited disease of Arabian foals in which T-lymphocytes and B-lymphocytes are absent. Foals appear normal at birth and grow free of disease for 3 to 8 weeks if adequate passive transfer of maternal antibody is obtained. Foals develop infection subsequent to catabolic elimination of maternal immunoglobulin. Clinical signs usually result from respiratory infection. Foals may initially respond to antimicrobial therapy; however, the severity of signs later worsens as more resistant infections develop. Foals generally die before 5 months of age.

INTERPRETATION OF LABORATORY DATA

Neutrophil count may be increased or decreased as a result of inflammation due to infection. Plasma fibrinogen concentration may be increased. Band neutrophils may be present. Complete blood count reveals a persistent lymphopenia (<1000/ml). Decreased B cell function decreases immunoglobulin production. However, immunoglobulins may be obtained from colostral absorption. As colostral titer decreases, immunoglobulin concentrations decrease. IgM may decrease first as less of it is obtained from colostrum. Decreased immunoglobulin concentrations may decrease globulin and total protein concentrations.

SIGNIFICANT DISEASES TO RULE OUT

- ◆ Pneumonia and septic arthritis that are not complicated by immunodeficiency are not accompanied by low concentrations of specific immunoglobulin isotypes and abnormal cell-mediated immune function.
- ◆ Selective IgM deficiency also results in recurring pneumonia but is not accompanied by lymphopenia and lymphoid hypoplasia.
- ◆ Other immune deficiency diseases are characterized by persistent or recurrent infections. Diagnosis is made by low to absent concentrations of specific immunoglobulins and abnormal cell-mediated immune function. These diseases include:
    Agammaglobulinemia
    Selective IgM deficiency
    Transient hypogammaglobulinemia
    Partial immunodeficiency
    Partial cell-mediated immunodeficiency

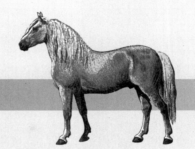

Signs

◆ Fever
◆ Coughing
◆ Tachypnea
◆ Nasal discharge

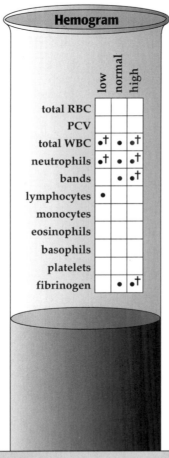

Serum Chemistry

	low	normal	high
CK			
AST			
SDH			
GGT			
bile acids			
bilirubin, total			
bilirubin, direct			
protein, total	•	•	
albumin			
globulin	•	•	
SUN			
creatinine			
glucose			
Ca			
P			
Na			
K			
Cl			
tCO$_2$			

Hemogram

	low	normal	high
total RBC			
PCV			
total WBC	•†	•	•†
neutrophils	•†	•	•†
bands		•	•†
lymphocytes	•		
monocytes			
eosinophils			
basophils			
platelets			
fibrinogen		•	•†

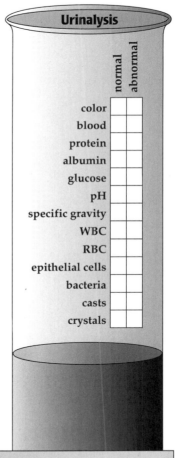

Urinalysis

	normal	abnormal
color		
blood		
protein		
albumin		
glucose		
pH		
specific gravity		
WBC		
RBC		
epithelial cells		
bacteria		
casts		
crystals		

Special Tests

◆ Serum immunoelectrophoresis (Veterinary Medical Research and Development, Inc., Pullman, WA) will reveal decreased IgM and IgG.
◆ Animals do not respond to vaccination with antibody titer.
◆ Histology reveals thymic hypoplasia and absence of germinal centers and follicles in lymph nodes.

• Changes caused by the disease itself
•† Changes secondary to dysfunction caused by the disease

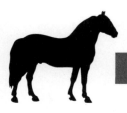

IgM Deficiency

This deficiency usually affects Arabian and Quarter horse breeds. Foals may present with severe pneumonia, enteritis, or arthritis and die by 1 year. A history of repeated, but antibiotic-responsive, infections is also common. Animals greater than 2 years of age present with respiratory signs, and some have been reported to develop malignant lymphoma. Animals may have signs of sepsis.

INTERPRETATION OF LABORATORY DATA

IgM deficiency is characterized by serum IgM concentration 2 standard deviations below age-matched controls with no other immune deficits. Lymphocyte counts are normal. IgG concentrations may be increased. Laboratory changes may reflect secondary infection.

SIGNIFICANT DISEASES TO RULE OUT

◆ Foals with failure of passive transfer have normal serum IgM concentrations.
◆ Combined immunodeficiency (CID) reveals absence of serum IgM, lymphopenia (<1000/ml), and hypoplasia of lymphoid tissues.

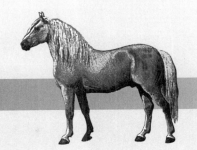

Signs

- Fever
- Coughing
- Tachypnea
- Nasal discharge

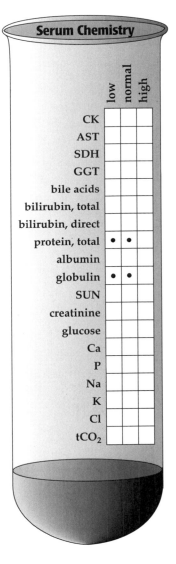

Serum Chemistry

	low	normal	high
CK			
AST			
SDH			
GGT			
bile acids			
bilirubin, total			
bilirubin, direct			
protein, total	•	•	
albumin			
globulin	•	•	
SUN			
creatinine			
glucose			
Ca			
P			
Na			
K			
Cl			
tCO$_2$			

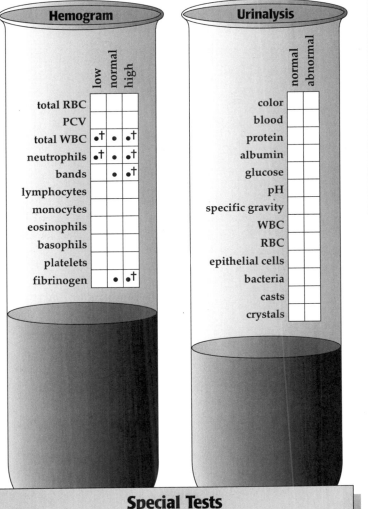

Hemogram

	low	normal	high
total RBC			
PCV			
total WBC	•†	•	•†
neutrophils	•†	•	•†
bands		•	•†
lymphocytes			
monocytes			
eosinophils			
basophils			
platelets			
fibrinogen		•	•†

Urinalysis

	normal	abnormal
color		
blood		
protein		
albumin		
glucose		
pH		
specific gravity		
WBC		
RBC		
epithelial cells		
bacteria		
casts		
crystals		

Special Tests

- Serum immunoelectrophoresis (Veterinary Medical Research and Development, Inc., Pullman, WA) will reveal decreased IgM; IgG concentration may be increased.

- Changes caused by the disease itself
- † Changes secondary to dysfunction caused by the disease

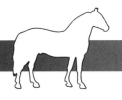

Renal Diseases

Acute renal failure

Chronic renal failure

Cystic calculi

Nephroliths and ureteral calculi

Uroperitoneum

Urinary tract infection

Urinary and renal neoplasia

Renal tubular acidosis

Spurious elevation of serum creatinine

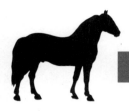

ACUTE RENAL FAILURE

Acute renal failure presents with a sudden development of uremia. This acute decrease in the glomerular filtration rate may occur because of hemodynamic changes and/or obstruction of renal tubules resulting from vasomotor nephropathy, toxic nephropathy, or interstitial nephritis. Renal failure is characterized by increased serum creatinine concentration with concurrent isosthenuria (specific gravity of 1.008 to 1.012); however, the diagnosis of renal failure is made only after consideration of clinical signs, state of hydration, and history of fluid or drug therapy. Horses are depressed and anorectic, and may be either anuric or polyuric.

INTERPRETATION OF LABORATORY DATA

The most common clinicopathologic findings in acute renal failure are hypochloridemia and hyponatremia, with hypocalcemia occurring infrequently. Acute renal failure may be polyuric or oliguric. Hyperkalemia is sometimes seen with oliguria, although this may be masked by the hypokalemia resulting from anorexia. Horses are isosthenuric and possibly acidotic. Results of the urinalysis will vary somewhat depending on the cause of renal failure. Aminoglycoside toxicity and pigment-induced nephropathy can cause tubular epithelial cell destruction with resulting increases in urine leukocytes, protein, casts, and blood. Urinary fractional excretion ratios of GGT greater than 25 indicate renal disease.

SIGNIFICANT DISEASES TO RULE OUT

- Prerenal azotemia will not result in isosthenuria.
- Pituitary adenoma does not cause azotemia. The urinalysis does not indicate inflammation.
- Chronic renal failure results from a slower, more progressive loss of nephrons over a longer period of time, resulting in weight loss and proteinuria. Histopathology of the kidney will reveal chronicity.

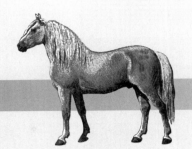

Signs

◆ Depression
◆ Anorexia
◆ Anuria or polyuria

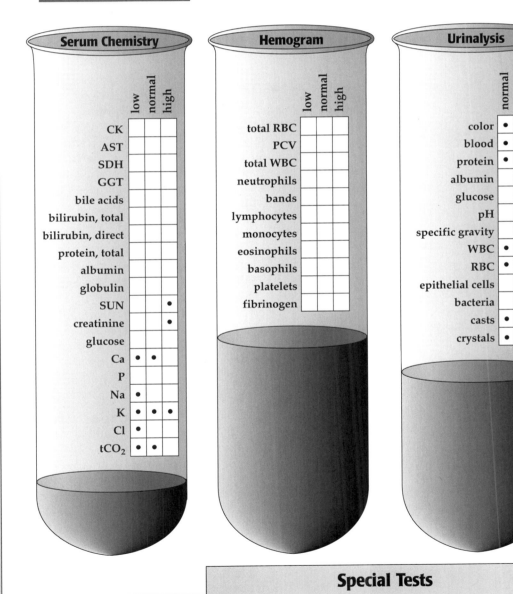

Serum Chemistry	low	normal	high
CK			
AST			
SDH			
GGT			
bile acids			
bilirubin, total			
bilirubin, direct			
protein, total			
albumin			
globulin			
SUN			•
creatinine			•
glucose			
Ca	•	•	
P			
Na	•		
K	•	•	•
Cl	•		
tCO$_2$	•	•	

Hemogram	low	normal	high
total RBC			
PCV			
total WBC			
neutrophils			
bands			
lymphocytes			
monocytes			
eosinophils			
basophils			
platelets			
fibrinogen			

Urinalysis	normal	abnormal
color	•	•
blood	•	•
protein	•	•
albumin		
glucose		
pH		
specific gravity		•
WBC	•	•
RBC	•	•
epithelial cells		
bacteria		
casts	•	•
crystals	•	•

Special Tests

◆ Urine GGT-creatinine ratio is greater than 25.

• Changes caused by the disease itself
•† Changes secondary to dysfunction caused by the disease

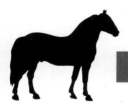

CHRONIC RENAL FAILURE

Chronic renal failure results from a slower, gradual loss of nephron function. It may follow a progressive tubulointerstitial or glomerular disease. Horses generally exhibit signs of depression, anorexia, weight loss, polyuria and polydipsia, foamy urine, and sometimes edema and colic. Dental tartar, melena, and oral ulcerations may occur in chronic cases. The same clinical considerations for diagnosis of acute renal failure apply to diagnosis of chronic renal failure.

INTERPRETATION OF LABORATORY DATA

Hypochloridemia and hyponatremia are common. Hypercalcemia frequently occurs, especially if the animal's diet is calcium rich. Serum phosphorus concentrations may vary inversely with the calcium concentration, but are typically not increased in equine chronic renal failure. There is usually moderate hyperkalemia and hypermagnesemia, though the hyperkalemia may be masked by the hypokalemia caused by anorexia. Moderate nonregenerative anemia may develop. The urine is isosthenuric and frequently contains protein and blood.

Proliferative glomerulonephritis is believed to result from the deposition of circulating antibody-antigen complexes in the glomeruli. Equine infectious anemia and possibly streptococcal antigens have been implicated. Laboratory findings include proteinuria, hypoproteinemia, and marked increase in the urine protein-creatinine ratio.

Acute extensive tubular necrosis or obstruction from emboli of *Actinobacillus equuli* may progress to chronic interstitial nephritis. Proteinuria and the nephrotic syndrome are not characteristic of this cause of renal failure.

SIGNIFICANT DISEASES TO RULE OUT

◆ Vitamin D (D_2 or D_3) toxicity from feed additives or plants (*Cestrum diurnum*) can induce renal failure. Mineralization in muscles, tendons, ligaments, vessel walls, and kidney results in clinical signs associated with disease of the respective tissues. Horses may exhibit weight loss, polydipsia, and polyuria. Laboratory findings are consistent with chronic renal failure, with the notable exception of increases in both serum calcium and phosphorus concentrations. Definitive diagnosis can be made by measurements of serum concentrations of vitamins D, D_2, and D_3.

◆ Pyelonephritis is an ascending lower urinary tract infection. Obstruction is the usual source of bacterial spread resulting in suppurative infection of the kidney. Pyuria, bacteriuria, mild proteinuria, hematuria, leukocytosis, hyperfibrinogenemia, and mild anemia may be present. The disease can progress to chronic renal failure.

◆ Pituitary adenoma does not cause azotemia or proteinuria.

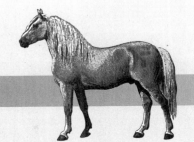

Signs

- ◆ Weight loss
- ◆ Polyuria
- ◆ Polydipsia
- ◆ Oral ulcerations
- ◆ Edema
- ◆ Foamy urine

Serum Chemistry

	low	normal	high
CK			
AST			
SDH			
GGT			
bile acids			
bilirubin, total			
bilirubin, direct			
protein, total	•	•	
albumin	•	•	
globulin	•	•	
SUN			•
creatinine			•
glucose			
Ca		•	•
P	•	•	
Na	•		
K	•	•	•
Cl	•		
tCO₂	•	•	

Hemogram

	low	normal	high
total RBC	•	•	
PCV	•	•	
total WBC			
neutrophils			
bands			
lymphocytes			
monocytes			
eosinophils			
basophils			
platelets			
fibrinogen			

Urinalysis

	normal	abnormal
color	•	•
blood	•	•
protein	•	•
albumin		
glucose		
pH		
specific gravity		•
WBC		
RBC		
epithelial cells		
bacteria		
casts		
crystals		

Special Tests

- ◆ Renal biopsy specimen may indicate degree of damage and fibrosis.
- ◆ Protein-creatinine ratio is greater than 2.
- ◆ Serum magnesium concentration may increase.

• Changes caused by the disease itself
•† Changes secondary to dysfunction caused by the disease

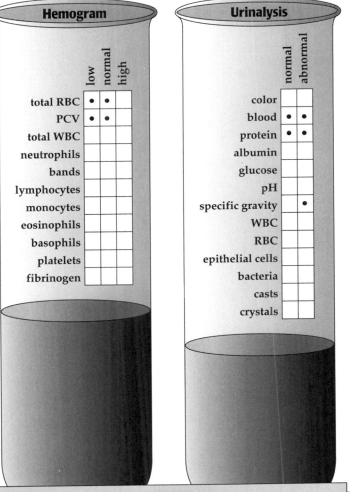

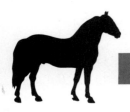

CYSTIC CALCULI

Equine cystic calculi are more common in adults and are usually composed of calcium carbonate or calcium phosphate salts. Clinical signs may include hematuria, stranguria, dysuria, pollakiuria, urine dribbling and scalding, and, less commonly, abdominal pain and loss of condition. Calculi may be palpated by rectal examination.

INTERPRETATION OF LABORATORY DATA

Laboratory findings are nonspecific and may only reflect a secondary bacterial infection with some hematuria and proteinuria. Urinalysis may reveal leukocytes, crystals, and bacteria.

SIGNIFICANT DISEASES TO RULE OUT

◆ Bacterial cystitis may be present as a primary disease without calculi or as a secondary complication of cystic calculi.
◆ Neurologic disease (e.g., cauda equina syndrome, herpesvirus) will usually exhibit other neurologic deficits.
◆ Neoplasia is definitively diagnosed by endoscopy and biopsy specimen interpretation.

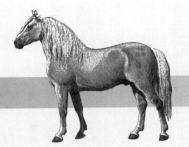

Signs

- ◆ Hematuria
- ◆ Stranguria
- ◆ Dysuria

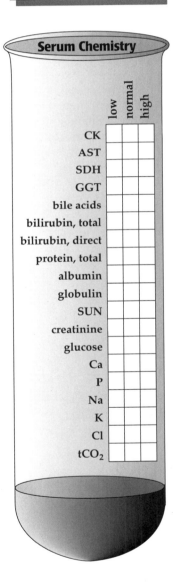

Serum Chemistry

	low	normal	high
CK			
AST			
SDH			
GGT			
bile acids			
bilirubin, total			
bilirubin, direct			
protein, total			
albumin			
globulin			
SUN			
creatinine			
glucose			
Ca			
P			
Na			
K			
Cl			
tCO$_2$			

Hemogram

	low	normal	high
total RBC			
PCV			
total WBC			
neutrophils			
bands			
lymphocytes			
monocytes			
eosinophils			
basophils			
platelets			
fibrinogen			

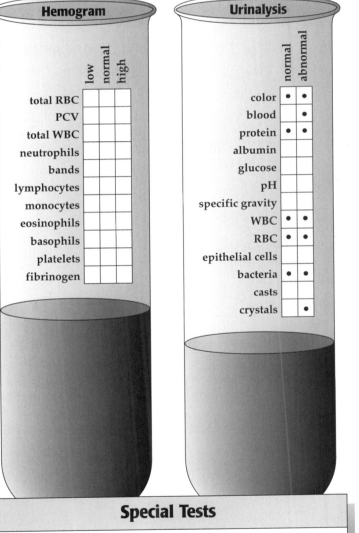

Urinalysis

	normal	abnormal
color	•	•
blood		•
protein	•	•
albumin		
glucose		
pH		
specific gravity		
WBC	•	•
RBC	•	•
epithelial cells		
bacteria	•	•
casts		
crystals		•

Special Tests

- ◆ Sonography may reveal calculus or granular obstruction.
- ◆ Endoscopy may visualize calculus.

• Changes caused by the disease itself
•† Changes secondary to dysfunction caused by the disease

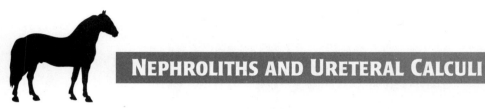

NEPHROLITHS AND URETERAL CALCULI

Nephroliths and ureteral calculi may be found in association with one or both kidneys or ureters and may cause complete, incomplete, or intermittent obstruction. In general, clinical signs are not severe; the animal is usually presented for weight loss and poor performance, rather than abdominal pain. Therefore the disease may progress to chronic renal failure before diagnosis. Calculi are reported more frequently in young adult Thoroughbred horses. The cause of stone formation is unknown.

INTERPRETATION OF LABORATORY DATA

If there is chronic bilateral obstruction, laboratory findings may reflect azotemia and isosthenuria of renal failure. Increased leukocytes, red cells, protein, isosthenuria, and crystals may be found on urinalysis. Calculi are usually composed of calcium carbonate or calcium phosphate.

SIGNIFICANT DISEASES TO RULE OUT

◆ Chronic renal failure will not reveal the presence of calculus.

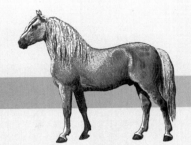

Signs

- ◆ Weight loss
- ◆ Poor performance
- ◆ Hematuria

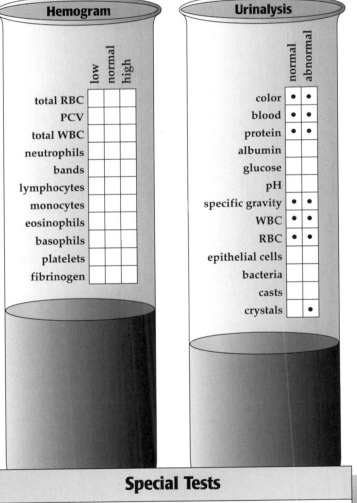

Serum Chemistry

	low	normal	high
CK			
AST			
SDH			
GGT			
bile acids			
bilirubin, total			
bilirubin, direct			
protein, total			
albumin			
globulin			
SUN		•	•
creatinine		•	•
glucose			
Ca			
P			
Na			
K			
Cl			
tCO$_2$			

Hemogram

	low	normal	high
total RBC			
PCV			
total WBC			
neutrophils			
bands			
lymphocytes			
monocytes			
eosinophils			
basophils			
platelets			
fibrinogen			

Urinalysis

	normal	abnormal
color	•	•
blood	•	•
protein	•	•
albumin		
glucose		
pH		
specific gravity	•	•
WBC	•	•
RBC	•	•
epithelial cells		
bacteria		
casts		
crystals		•

Special Tests

- ◆ Sonography of kidney may reveal calculi.
- ◆ Renal biopsy specimen will indicate obstructive damage.
- ◆ Rectal examination may reveal distended ureter/kidney.

- • Changes caused by the disease itself
- •† Changes secondary to dysfunction caused by the disease

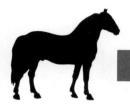

UROPERITONEUM

The most common cause of urine leakage into the abdomen is a ruptured urinary bladder, but urine may also leak from the ureters, urachus, and urethra. Uroperitoneum is most common in neonatal male foals and is frequently associated with parturition. Developmental anomalies, trauma, recumbency, and rupture of umbilical/urachal abscesses and necrosis have also been reported as predisposing causes. Rupture is uncommon in adult horses, but may occur in postpartum mares or as a sequela to obstruction or neurologic disease. Animals exhibit signs of stranguria, incontinence, depression, colic, increasing abdominal distention and pain, tachycardia, tachypnea, and abnormal urination.

INTERPRETATION OF LABORATORY DATA

The large volume of dilute urine that is low in sodium and chloride and high in potassium equilibrates across the large surface area of peritoneum. Serum electrolyte abnormalities are marked and include hyponatremia in the presence of normal hydration, hypochloremia, hyperkalemia, and mild metabolic acidosis (decreased total CO_2). The ratio of abdominal fluid to serum creatinine is usually > 2, but the serum creatinine and SUN concentrations will increase with time. Dehydration leads to an increased PCV, and the leukocyte count may increase. In foals, the serum glucose concentration may be low because of anorexia.

SIGNIFICANT DISEASES TO RULE OUT

- Ureteral or urethral obstruction without rupture may present with some lumbar pain and oliguria or anuria without uroperitoneum.
- Neonatal isoerythrolysis causes anemia and hemoglobinemia.
- Meconium impaction can be identified by digital palpation or abdominal radiographs. Azotemia, hyponatremia, and hyperkalemia are not present.
- Septicemia does not cause hyponatremia and hyperkalemia. The neutrophil count is often decreased, with an increased number of band neutrophils.
- Strangulating obstruction does not cause hyponatremia and hyperkalemia.

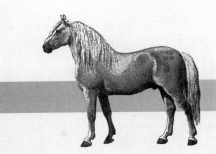

Signs

- Depression
- Colic
- Abdominal distention
- Stranguria
- Incontinence
- Weakness
- Dyspnea

Serum Chemistry

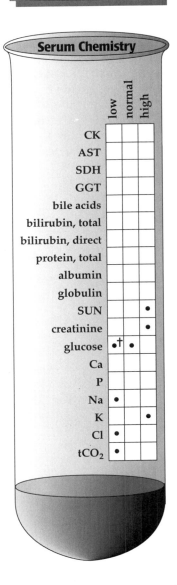

	low	normal	high
CK			
AST			
SDH			
GGT			
bile acids			
bilirubin, total			
bilirubin, direct			
protein, total			
albumin			
globulin			
SUN			•
creatinine			•
glucose	•†	•	
Ca			
P			
Na	•		
K			•
Cl	•		
tCO₂	•		

Hemogram

	low	normal	high
total RBC		•	•
PCV		•	•
total WBC	•	•	
neutrophils			
bands			
lymphocytes			
monocytes			
eosinophils			
basophils			
platelets			
fibrinogen			

Urinalysis

	normal	abnormal
color		
blood		
protein		
albumin		
glucose		
pH		
specific gravity	•	•
WBC		
RBC		
epithelial cells		
bacteria		
casts		
crystals		

Special Tests

- Peritoneal fluid creatinine to serum creatinine concentration ratio will be ≥ 2:1.
- Contrast radiography and ultrasonography may detect the location of the defect.

- Changes caused by the disease itself
- † Changes secondary to dysfunction caused by the disease

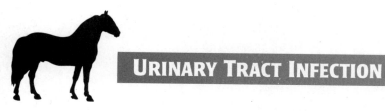

URINARY TRACT INFECTION

Bacterial cystitis may be associated with urine stasis, prolonged catheterization, calculi or neoplasia, neurologic disease, and ascending infection from reproductive problems such as dystocia. The animal may exhibit dysuria, stranguria, or pollakiuria with blood-tinged urine.

INTERPRETATION OF LABORATORY DATA

A clean-catch or catheterized urine specimen should be analyzed and cultured. If analysis and culture cannot be performed immediately, the specimen should be refrigerated. The presence of significant bacteria and leukocytes (> 5 leukocytes/HPF) is indicative of a urinary tract infection. Culture counts of $\geq 10 \times 10^3$ CFU bacteria/ml from a catheterized specimen are significant. Common bacterial isolates are *E. coli*, *Proteus, Klebsiella, Pseudomonas, Streptococcus*, and *Staphylococcus*.

SIGNIFICANT DISEASES TO RULE OUT

- Pyelonephritis reveals mild proteinuria and hematuria similar to that of a urinary tract infection, but there is also leukocytosis and hyperfibrinogenemia. A mild anemia may be present. A dilated renal pelvis may be detected with ultrasonography.

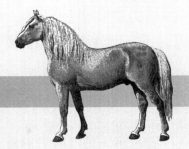

Signs

- ◆ Dysuria
- ◆ Stranguria
- ◆ Pollakiuria

Serum Chemistry

	low	normal	high
CK			
AST			
SDH			
GGT			
bile acids			
bilirubin, total			
bilirubin, direct			
protein, total			
albumin			
globulin			
SUN			
creatinine			
glucose			
Ca			
P			
Na			
K			
Cl			
tCO$_2$			

Hemogram

	low	normal	high
total RBC			
PCV			
total WBC			
neutrophils			
bands			
lymphocytes			
monocytes			
eosinophils			
basophils			
platelets			
fibrinogen			

Urinalysis

	normal	abnormal
color	●	●
blood	●	●
protein		●
albumin		
glucose		
pH		
specific gravity		
WBC		●
RBC	●	●
epithelial cells		
bacteria		●
casts		
crystals		

Special Tests

- ◆ Urine culture should be performed to identify causative agent and proper antimicrobial therapy.

- ● Changes caused by the disease itself
- ●† Changes secondary to dysfunction caused by the disease

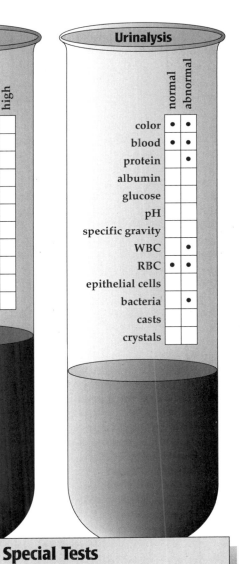

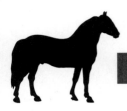

URINARY AND RENAL NEOPLASIA

Equine bladder tumors are uncommon, and occur in middle-aged to older horses. Squamous-cell carcinoma, rather than transitional cell carcinoma, is most common. Hematuria, stranguria, dysuria, weight loss, and depression are clinical signs. Rectal examination or ultrasonography may reveal a mass.

INTERPRETATION OF LABORATORY DATA

Urinalysis frequently reveals hematuria, proteinuria, and pyuria consistent with a secondary cystitis. Examination of urine sediment for the presence of neoplastic cells should be performed, but a diagnosis by urine cytology alone is uncommon. Neoplastic cells may not exfoliate, or they may be too deteriorated for identification. In long-standing cases a nonregenerative anemia may develop.

SIGNIFICANT DISEASES TO RULE OUT

◆ Cystitis responds favorably to antibiotic therapy.
◆ Cystic calculi may be differentiated by detection of calculus.
◆ Neurologic disease with cystitis will usually present with other neurologic deficits.

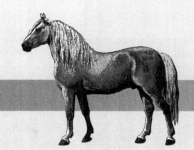

Signs

- Hematuria
- Dysuria
- Weight loss

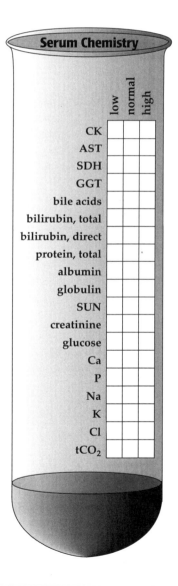

Serum Chemistry

	low	normal	high
CK			
AST			
SDH			
GGT			
bile acids			
bilirubin, total			
bilirubin, direct			
protein, total			
albumin			
globulin			
SUN			
creatinine			
glucose			
Ca			
P			
Na			
K			
Cl			
tCO$_2$			

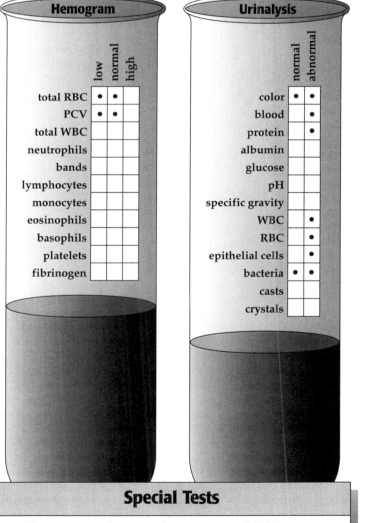

Hemogram

	low	normal	high
total RBC	•	•	
PCV	•	•	
total WBC			
neutrophils			
bands			
lymphocytes			
monocytes			
eosinophils			
basophils			
platelets			
fibrinogen			

Urinalysis

	normal	abnormal
color	•	•
blood		•
protein		•
albumin		
glucose		
pH		
specific gravity		
WBC		•
RBC		•
epithelial cells		•
bacteria	•	•
casts		
crystals		

Special Tests

- Ultrasonography may detect renal or bladder masses or abnormalities.
- Endoscopy may reveal bladder mass.
- Biopsy may be necessary to confirm neoplasia.

- Changes caused by the disease itself
- † Changes secondary to dysfunction caused by the disease

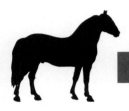

RENAL TUBULAR ACIDOSIS

Renal tubular acidosis (RTA) occurs with tubular loss of bicarbonate from plasma and replacement by chloride. With Type 1 RTA, the distal renal tubule fails to secrete hydrogen ions. In Type 2, the proximal tubule inadequately resorbs bicarbonate. Animals exhibit a resultant hyperchloremic acidosis. RTA can occur primarily or secondarily to another systemic disease. Clinical signs in horses include anorexia, depression, weight loss, and weakness.

INTERPRETATION OF LABORATORY DATA

Animals develop hyperchloremic acidosis as a result of tubular loss of bicarbonate and replacement by chloride. In Type 1 RTA, horses cannot acidify urine and have a persistently alkaline urine. With Type 2 RTA, horses are capable of acidifying urine when the acidosis is marked. The glomerular filtration rate is usually normal, so azotemia and uremia are not usually present, though horses may be isosthenuric. Horses may be hypokalemic as a result of anorexia and renal loss. A neutrophilic leukocytosis is sometimes seen, particularly if the RTA is secondary to another systemic disease.

SIGNIFICANT DISEASES TO RULE OUT

◆ Renal failure will present with azotemia and isosthenuria.

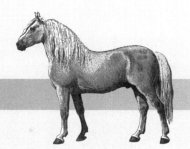

Signs

- ◆ Anorexia
- ◆ Depression
- ◆ Weight loss
- ◆ Weakness

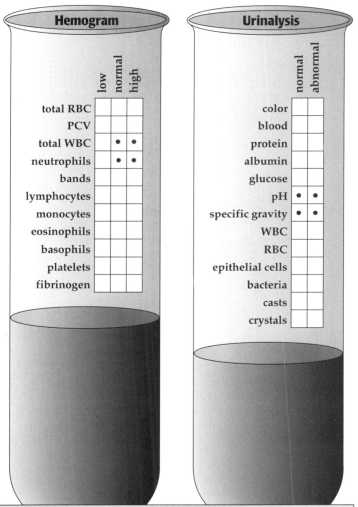

Serum Chemistry

	low	normal	high
CK			
AST			
SDH			
GGT			
bile acids			
bilirubin, total			
bilirubin, direct			
protein, total			
albumin			
globulin			
SUN			
creatinine			
glucose			
Ca			
P			
Na			
K	●	●	
Cl			●
tCO₂	●		

Hemogram

	low	normal	high
total RBC			
PCV			
total WBC		●	●
neutrophils		●	●
bands			
lymphocytes			
monocytes			
eosinophils			
basophils			
platelets			
fibrinogen			

Urinalysis

	normal	abnormal
color		
blood		
protein		
albumin		
glucose		
pH	●	●
specific gravity	●	●
WBC		
RBC		
epithelial cells		
bacteria		
casts		
crystals		

Special Tests

- ◆ Bicarbonate loading will produce an alkaline urine in the face of systemic acidosis with Type 2 RTA but no increase in urinary pH with Type 1 RTA.

● Changes caused by the disease itself

●† Changes secondary to dysfunction caused by the disease

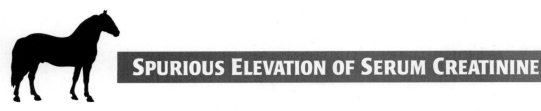

SPURIOUS ELEVATION OF SERUM CREATININE

Serum creatinine concentration in newborn foals sometimes is higher than that of the mare for the first 3 days of life. Rarely in a healthy term foal, the serum creatinine concentration may be 5 to 10 times normal. Serum creatinine concentrations in premature foals commonly are increased. There are no abnormal clinical signs associated with these elevations. The cause is unknown. However, the inability to equilibrate across the placental membranes (healthy or diseased) has been suggested.

INTERPRETATION OF LABORATORY DATA

The serum creatinine concentration is increased but serum electrolyte concentration, urinalysis, and all other values are normal. Urine specific gravity in a foal is normally less than 1.010. The serum creatinine concentration decreases rapidly in a few days.

DISEASES TO RULE OUT

- ◆ Uroperitoneum will result in hyponatremia, hypokalemia, and hypochloremia. Abdominal fluid creatinine concentration will be greater than 2 times serum concentration.
- ◆ Renal failure will also frequently cause abnormalities in serum electrolytes and urinalysis. There also will be clinical signs of disease, including lethargy and decreased suckling.
- ◆ Prerenal azotemia will result in clinical signs of dehydration.

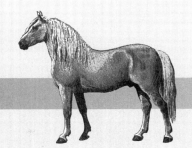

Signs

◆ Normal behavior

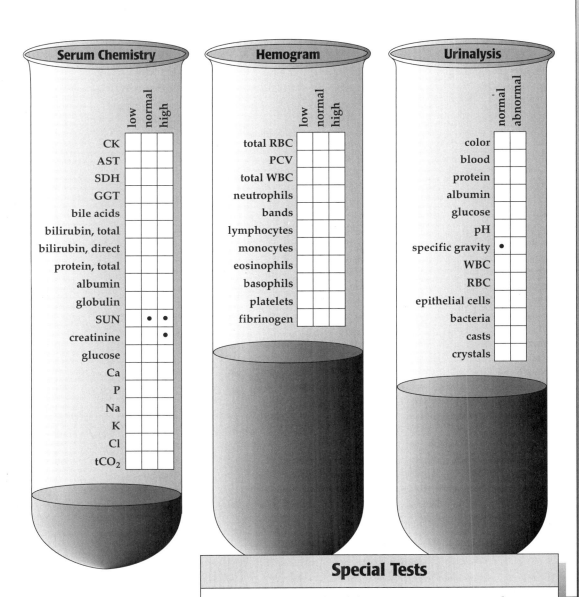

Serum Chemistry	low	normal	high
CK			
AST			
SDH			
GGT			
bile acids			
bilirubin, total			
bilirubin, direct			
protein, total			
albumin			
globulin			
SUN		●	●
creatinine			●
glucose			
Ca			
P			
Na			
K			
Cl			
tCO₂			

Hemogram	low	normal	high
total RBC			
PCV			
total WBC			
neutrophils			
bands			
lymphocytes			
monocytes			
eosinophils			
basophils			
platelets			
fibrinogen			

Urinalysis	normal	abnormal
color		
blood		
protein		
albumin		
glucose		
pH		
specific gravity	●	
WBC		
RBC		
epithelial cells		
bacteria		
casts		
crystals		

Special Tests

◆ Results of all other laboratory tests are normal unless there is concurrent disease.

● Changes caused by the disease itself
●† Changes secondary to dysfunction caused by the disease

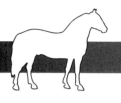

Hepatic Diseases

Acute hepatitis

Chronic active hepatitis

Pyrrolizidine alkaloid toxicity

Cholelithiasis

Hyperlipemia

Tyzzer's disease

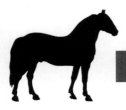

ACUTE HEPATITIS

Infectious, toxic, and undefined etiologies may cause acute hepatitis. Because the liver has great reserve capacity, clinical signs are not apparent until greater than 50% of the hepatic mass is destroyed. Clinical signs may then appear suddenly, with horses appearing depressed, anorectic, and icteric. Photosensitization, diarrhea, and clotting abnormalities, indicated by excessive bleeding, may occur. Neurologic signs resulting from hypoglycemia and hepatic encephalopathy can be most severe in horses with acute fulminant liver disease. Signs of endotoxemia (e.g., tachycardia, fever, and hyperemic mucous membranes) may be present.

INTERPRETATION OF LABORATORY DATA

Increases in serum SDH and AST activities are indicative of acute hepatocellular injury. In general, the increase in enzyme activity correlates with the number of hepatocytes affected. The resulting cholestasis from this injury manifests as hyperbilirubinemia. Increase in serum GGT activity occurs secondary to hepatocyte swelling. Direct (conjugated) bilirubin usually ranges from 15% to 40% of total. As the hepatic disease progresses, liver function becomes compromised, which can be detected by increases in serum bile acid concentration, prolonged BSP clearance, and decreased glucose and SUN concentrations. Coagulation tests may become prolonged with increasing liver failure. Anorexia can lead to hypokalemia. The CBC may reflect neutrophilia or, if endotoxemia occurs, a neutropenia with increased band neutrophils and toxic changes.

SIGNIFICANT DISEASES TO RULE OUT

- Tyzzer's disease is a highly fatal disease affecting foals at 1 to 6 weeks of age. Sudden onset of fever, depression, and increase in hepatocellular enzyme activity leads to a comatose state and usually death.
- Cerebral disease alone will not present with abnormal laboratory data of liver disease.
- Hemolysis is associated with a moderate to marked anemia.

Signs

- ◆ Depression
- ◆ Anorexia
- ◆ ± Icterus
- ◆ ± Photosensitization
- ◆ ± Diarrhea
- ◆ ± Hemorrhage
- ◆ ± Encephalopathy

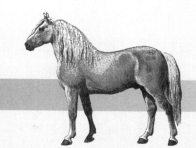

Serum Chemistry

	low	normal	high
CK			
AST			•
SDH			•
GGT		•	•
bile acids		•	•
bilirubin, total		•	•
bilirubin, direct		•	•
protein, total			
albumin			
globulin			
SUN	•	•	
creatinine			
glucose	•	•	
Ca			
P			
Na			
K	•†	•	
Cl			
tCO₂			

Hemogram

	low	normal	high
total RBC			
PCV			
total WBC	•	•	•
neutrophils	•	•	•
bands		•	•
lymphocytes			
monocytes			
eosinophils			
basophils			
platelets			
fibrinogen			

Urinalysis

	normal	abnormal
color		
blood		
protein		
albumin		
glucose		
pH		
specific gravity		
WBC		
RBC		
epithelial cells		
bacteria		
casts		
crystals		

Special Tests

- ◆ BSP may be prolonged with severe hepatic disease.
- ◆ APTT and OSPT are prolonged in severe cases.
- ◆ Liver biopsy will reveal characteristics of inflammation and hepatocellular damage.
- ◆ Culture of liver biopsy sometimes reveals bacterial etiology.

- • Changes caused by the disease itself
- •† Changes secondary to dysfunction caused by the disease

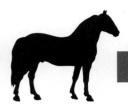

CHRONIC ACTIVE HEPATITIS

Many causes of acute hepatic failure can progress to chronic active hepatitis. In addition to signs seen in horses with acute hepatitis, such as depression, anorexia, photosensitization, diarrhea, excessive bleeding, encephalopathy, and sometimes icterus, these animals may present with chronic, progressive weight loss.

INTERPRETATION OF LABORATORY DATA

Serum liver enzyme activities can be variably increased, but in cases with marked hepatic fibrosis, enzyme activity may be within reference range, and SUN and albumin concentrations may be decreased. Serum globulins may be normal or increased. Liver function tests (bile acids, BSP) usually indicate decreased function. With diminishing hepatic function, serum glucose concentration and concentrations of coagulation factors drop, and OSPT and APTT become prolonged. Affected animals frequently have indications of cholestasis such that greater than 25% of total bilirubin is direct (conjugated). Clinical signs and laboratory data of hepatic failure with characteristic histopathologic lesions of the liver are diagnostic. There may be neutrophilia or neutropenia with a left shift if endotoxemia occurs. With increasing chronicity of disease, a nonregenerative anemia and hyperfibrinogenemia can develop. Anorexia can lead to hypokalemia.

SIGNIFICANT DISEASES TO RULE OUT

- Pyrrolizidine alkaloid toxicity can be distinguished by the classic histopathology with which it is associated. In cases where serum chemistries are not diagnostic of hepatic failure, liver function tests (bile acids, BSP) may aid in diagnosis.
- Hemolysis is associated with a moderate to marked anemia.
- Acute hepatitis is differentiated by duration of signs and liver biopsy findings. Weight loss is not a key sign in acute hepatitis.

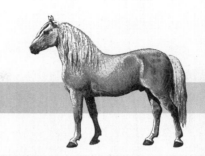

Signs

- ◆ Depression
- ◆ Anorexia
- ◆ ± Icterus
- ◆ ± Photosensitization
- ◆ ± Diarrhea
- ◆ ± Hemorrhage
- ◆ ± Encephalopathy
- ◆ Chronic weight loss

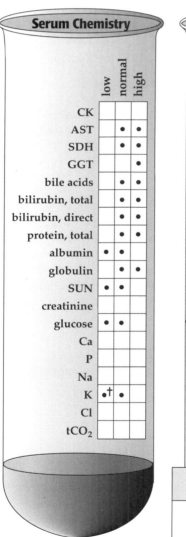

Serum Chemistry

	low	normal	high
CK			
AST		•	•
SDH		•	•
GGT			•
bile acids		•	•
bilirubin, total		•	•
bilirubin, direct		•	•
protein, total		•	•
albumin	•	•	
globulin		•	•
SUN	•	•	
creatinine			
glucose	•	•	
Ca			
P			
Na			
K	•†	•	
Cl			
tCO₂			

Hemogram

	low	normal	high
total RBC	•	•	
PCV	•	•	
total WBC	•	•	•
neutrophils	•	•	•
bands		•	•
lymphocytes			
monocytes			
eosinophils			
basophils			
platelets			
fibrinogen		•	•

Urinalysis

	normal	abnormal
color		
blood		
protein		
albumin		
glucose		
pH		
specific gravity		
WBC		
RBC		
epithelial cells		
bacteria		
casts		
crystals		

Special Tests

- ◆ Liver biopsy reveals classic histopathology diagnostic for chronic hepatitis.
- ◆ BSP clearance is prolonged.
- ◆ APTT and OSPT may be prolonged.
- ◆ Culture of liver biopsy sometimes reveals bacterial etiology.

• Changes caused by the disease itself
•† Changes secondary to dysfunction caused by the disease

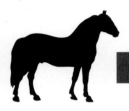

PYRROLIZIDINE ALKALOID TOXICITY

Pyrrolizidine alkaloid toxicity most commonly presents as a chronic and progressive hepatopathy, but an acute hepatic intoxication can occur. This disease is caused by ingestion of plants (*Amsinckia intermedia*, *Crotalaria* spp., *Heliotropium europeum*, *Echium lycopsis*, *Senecio*) found in certain geographic areas. Although the clinical signs of pyrrolizidine alkaloid toxicity may not develop for several months, the animal usually presents acutely. Signs of encephalopathy include head-pressing, blindness, and somnolence. Icterus and photosensitization are variable. Horses are in poor condition, and may also present with gastrointestinal signs of anorexia, diarrhea, and decreased borborygmi.

INTERPRETATION OF LABORATORY DATA

Depending on the stage of the disease, laboratory data indicate progressive hepatocellular and cholestatic liver disease. The more chronic, end-stage presentation may demonstrate higher activities of GGT, no increases in SDH and AST activity, decreased SUN and albumin, prolonged APTT and OSPT, and hypoglycemia. Serum globulins may be increased. Liver function tests (bile acids, BSP) may indicate decreased function. Anorexia can lead to hypokalemia. In cases of acute intoxication, SDH and AST serum enzyme activities may be increased. There may be neutrophilia or neutropenia with a left shift if endotoxemia occurs. With increasing chronicity of disease, a nonregenerative anemia and hyperfibrinogenemia can develop. A liver biopsy specimen will reveal classic histopathology of megalocytes, bile duct proliferation, and fibrosis.

SIGNIFICANT DISEASES TO RULE OUT

◆ A liver biopsy specimen may be necessary to differentiate chronic active hepatitis.

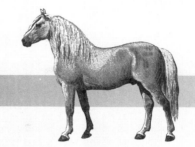

Signs

- ◆ Anorexia
- ◆ Weight loss
- ◆ Head-pressing
- ◆ Somnolence
- ◆ Diarrhea
- ◆ ± Icterus

Serum Chemistry

	low	normal	high
CK			
AST		•	•
SDH		•	•
GGT		•	•
bile acids		•	•
bilirubin, total		•	•
bilirubin, direct		•	•
protein, total			
albumin	•	•	
globulin		•	•
SUN	•	•	
creatinine			
glucose			
Ca			
P			
Na			
K	•†	•	
Cl			
tCO$_2$			

Hemogram

	low	normal	high
total RBC	•	•	
PCV	•	•	
total WBC	•	•	•
neutrophils	•	•	•
bands		•	•
lymphocytes			
monocytes			
eosinophils			
basophils			
platelets			
fibrinogen		•	•

Urinalysis

	normal	abnormal
color		
blood		
protein		
albumin		
glucose		
pH		
specific gravity		
WBC		
RBC		
epithelial cells		
bacteria		
casts		
crystals		

Special Tests

- ◆ Biopsy of liver reveals classic histopathology including megalocytes, fibrosis, and bile duct proliferation.
- ◆ BSP clearance is prolonged.
- ◆ APTT and OSPT may be prolonged.

- • Changes caused by the disease itself
- •† Changes secondary to dysfunction caused by the disease

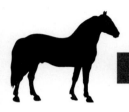

CHOLELITHIASIS

Choleliths are found more frequently in horses older than 9 years of age. Clinical signs include weight loss, abdominal pain, icterus, and intermittent fever. Horses with long-standing cases of cholelithiasis may exhibit encephalopathy. The cause of cholelith formation in horses is not known.

INTERPRETATION OF LABORATORY DATA

Horses have hyperbilirubinemia with increased conjugated bilirubin, and serum GGT activity is markedly increased. Bile acids concentration is frequently increased. SDH and AST activities are also increased secondarily and to a lesser degree. Laboratory findings consistent with inflammation—leukocytosis, anemia of chronic disease, hyperproteinemia, hyperglobulinemia, and hyperfibrinogenemia—are present. SUN is usually decreased and liver function tests (bile acids, BSP) indicate reduced function. If anorexia develops, hypokalemia follows. Glucose concentration may be decreased, and APTT and OSPT may be prolonged. Ultrasonography may reveal dilated bile ducts and hyperechoic regions diagnostic of choleliths. A liver biopsy specimen will likely reveal bile stasis and canalicular plugs with mild fibrosis.

SIGNIFICANT DISEASES TO RULE OUT

- Hepatitis causes increased serum SDH and AST activities to a greater degree than GGT activity.
- Hemolysis is associated with a moderate to marked anemia.
- Chronic recurrent colic will present without marked abnormalities in serum chemistries.

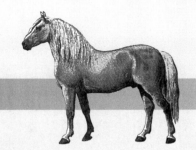

Signs

- ◆ Abdominal pain
- ◆ Icterus
- ◆ Fever

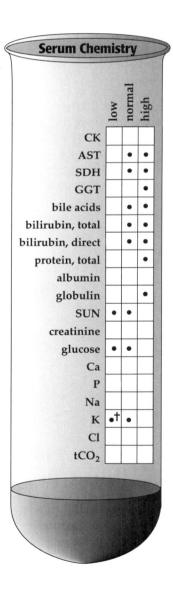

Serum Chemistry

	low	normal	high
CK			
AST		•	•
SDH		•	•
GGT			•
bile acids		•	•
bilirubin, total		•	•
bilirubin, direct		•	•
protein, total			•
albumin			
globulin			•
SUN	•	•	
creatinine			
glucose	•	•	
Ca			
P			
Na			
K	•†	•	
Cl			
tCO$_2$			

Hemogram

	low	normal	high
total RBC	•	•	
PCV	•	•	
total WBC		•	•
neutrophils		•	•
bands		•	•
lymphocytes			
monocytes			
eosinophils			
basophils			
platelets			
fibrinogen			•

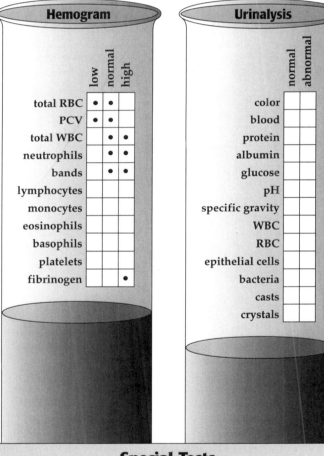

Urinalysis

	normal	abnormal
color		
blood		
protein		
albumin		
glucose		
pH		
specific gravity		
WBC		
RBC		
epithelial cells		
bacteria		
casts		
crystals		

Special Tests

- ◆ Ultrasonography of liver may reveal choleliths.
- ◆ BSP clearance may be prolonged.
- ◆ Liver biopsy can aid in differentiating etiology of liver disease.
- ◆ APTT and OSPT may be prolonged.
- ◆ Culture of liver biopsy may reveal bacterial infection.

• Changes caused by the disease itself
•† Changes secondary to dysfunction caused by the disease

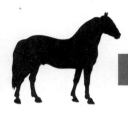

HYPERLIPEMIA

Hyperlipemia syndrome is primarily a disease of obese ponies and is more common during pregnancy and lactation. Donkeys and, less frequently, horses may be affected. The onset of disease has been associated with stress, decreased feed intake, and an insulin resistance resulting in mobilization of fat. Anorexia, diarrhea, dullness, and lethargy may progress to more severe depression and eventual death.

INTERPRETATION OF LABORATORY DATA

Animals are hypertriglyceridemic, hypoglycemic, and acidotic with grossly lipemic plasma. Liver function (bile acids, BSP) may be compromised, APTT and OSPT may be prolonged, and hepatocellular enzyme activities (AST, SDH) may be increased. Increased creatinine, isosthenuria, and metabolic acidosis (decreased tCO_2) may occur secondary to renal disease. Anorexia can lead to hypokalemia. Animals may become neutropenic with increased band neutrophils. Pancreatitis has been reported in some cases. Chemistry assays determined by optical density and some colorimetric methods may be affected by lipemic serum.

SIGNIFICANT DISEASES TO RULE OUT

◆ Starvation may cause a mild hyperlipemia without laboratory indications of liver or renal disease.
◆ Pituitary adenoma (equine Cushing's disease) in older horses and ponies causes hyperlipemia, but does not result in signs of acute illness. Liver enzyme activities may be mildly increased without changes in liver function.

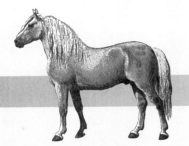

Signs

- ◆ Anorexia
- ◆ Diarrhea
- ◆ Lethargy

Serum Chemistry

	low	normal	high
CK			
AST		•	•
SDH		•	•
GGT		•	•
bile acids		•	•
bilirubin, total		•	•
bilirubin, direct		•	•
protein, total			
albumin			
globulin			
SUN	•	•	•†
creatinine		•	•†
glucose	•		
Ca			
P			
Na			
K	•†	•	
Cl			
tCO₂	•		

Hemogram

	low	normal	high
total RBC			
PCV			
total WBC	•	•	
neutrophils	•	•	
bands		•	•
lymphocytes			
monocytes			
eosinophils			
basophils			
platelets			
fibrinogen			

Urinalysis

	normal	abnormal
color		
blood		
protein		
albumin		
glucose		
pH		
specific gravity	•	•
WBC		
RBC		
epithelial cells		
bacteria		
casts		
crystals		

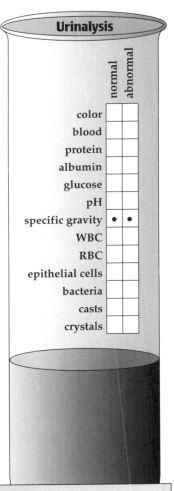

Special Tests

- ◆ Plasma triglyceride levels are increased.
- ◆ Plasma is grossly lipemic.
- ◆ APTT and OSPT may be prolonged with severe disease.
- ◆ BSP clearance may be prolonged.

•   Changes caused by the disease itself
•† Changes secondary to dysfunction caused by the disease

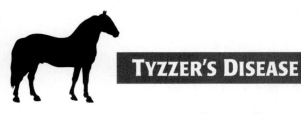

TYZZER'S DISEASE

Tyzzer's disease is acute multifocal hepatitis due to infection with *Clostridium piliformis*, occurring in foals 7 to 42 days of age. Clinical signs include depression and fever with rapid progression to coma and death. Icterus is a variable clinical sign. Sudden death may be the only clinical sign. Natural infection is thought to occur by oral ingestion, but predisposing factors are poorly understood.

INTERPRETATION OF LABORATORY DATA

Serum concentrations of hepatocellular enzymes (GGT, AST, SDH), bile acids, and bilirubin concentrations are usually increased. Complete blood count and neutrophil count may be increased or decreased. Band neutrophil count may be increased.

SIGNIFICANT DISEASES TO RULE OUT

◆ Neonatal isoerythrolysis usually occurs in younger foals and is accompanied by anemia.
◆ Sepsis usually occurs in younger foals. Liver function tests are normal.

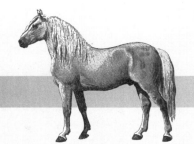

Signs

- ◆ Depression
- ◆ Fever
- ◆ ± Icterus
- ◆ Coma
- ◆ Death

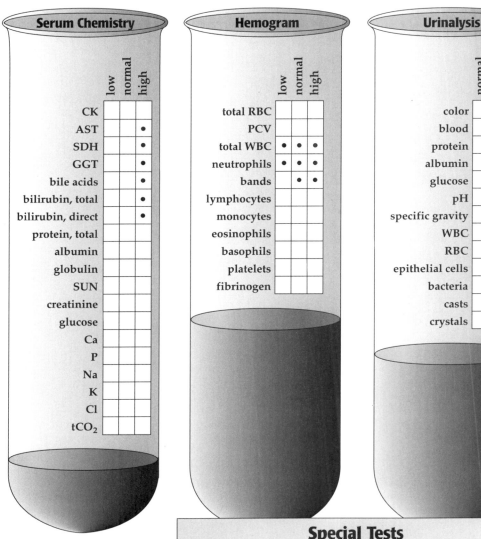

Serum Chemistry

	low	normal	high
CK			
AST			•
SDH			•
GGT			•
bile acids			•
bilirubin, total			•
bilirubin, direct			•
protein, total			
albumin			
globulin			
SUN			
creatinine			
glucose			
Ca			
P			
Na			
K			
Cl			
tCO$_2$			

Hemogram

	low	normal	high
total RBC			
PCV			
total WBC	•	•	•
neutrophils	•	•	•
bands		•	•
lymphocytes			
monocytes			
eosinophils			
basophils			
platelets			
fibrinogen			

Urinalysis

	normal	abnormal
color		
blood		
protein		
albumin		
glucose		
pH		
specific gravity		
WBC		
RBC		
epithelial cells		
bacteria		
casts		
crystals		

Special Tests

- ◆ Histopathology of liver reveals classic lesions and bacterial rods within hepatocytes.

- • Changes caused by the disease itself
- •† Changes secondary to dysfunction caused by the disease

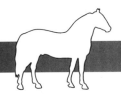

Central Nervous System Diseases

Viral encephalitides

Leukoencephalomalacia

Brain and spinal abscesses

Equine protozoal myeloencephalitis

Meningitis

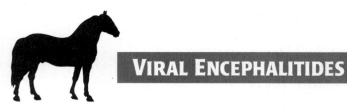

VIRAL ENCEPHALITIDES

Encephalomyelitis caused by viral agents includes western (WEE) and eastern (EEE) encephalomyelitis, equine herpesvirus 1 myeloencephalitis (EHV-1), equine infectious anemia, and rabies.

Clinical signs of western and eastern encephalomyelitis are usually first recognized as fever and changes in behavior. This may progress to hyperesthesia, excitability, and anorexia. Progressive dementia, circling, signs of cranial nerve disease, and blindness frequently result.

EHV-1 infrequently causes fever, paresis, and ataxia of trunk (particularly of the pelvic limbs).

The clinical indications of EIA and rabies are variable signs relating to diffuse CNS disease, ranging from lameness to depression to mania to sudden death.

INTERPRETATION OF LABORATORY DATA

Hyperglycemia has been associated with cerebral diseases.

With EEE and WEE, lymphopenia and neutropenia can be mild, progressing to profound, depending on the stage of the disease. Cerebrospinal fluid (CSF) analysis reveals an increased protein and cell count, which consists predominantly of neutrophils in the early stages and lymphocytes later in the disease. A fourfold increase from acute to convalescent serum titers by hemagglutination-inhibition or complement fixation indicates disease. Virus and vaccine titers can be distinguished by use of an ELISA or comparison of EEE and WEE titers. Fresh or frozen brain tissue is best for virus isolation. Histopathologic examination of the brain will reveal characteristic supportive lesions.

In EHV-1-induced CNS disease, isolation of virus from nasopharyngeal swabs or blood, a fourfold increase in serum-neutralizing or complement-fixation serum titers, or CSF antibody titers indicate disease. CSF appears xanthochromic with increased protein concentration.

With rabies, CSF analysis may be normal or reveal a mildly increased protein and cell count. Fluorescent antibody test of the brain (preferably hippocampus and cerebellum) is the diagnostic test.

SIGNIFICANT DISEASES TO RULE OUT

- Hepatoencephalopathy can be diagnosed by serum chemistries. Protozoal myeloencephalitis is diagnosed by Western blot analysis of CSF (University of Kentucky).
- Verminous or bacterial meningoencephalomyelitis is suspected when viral and protozoal titers are negative.
- Leukoencephalomalacia undergoes a rapid progression to death.
- Brain trauma may present with evidence of hemorrhage in CSF.

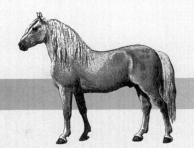

Signs

- ◆ Fever
- ◆ Behavior change
- ◆ Circling
- ◆ Ataxia
- ◆ Blindness

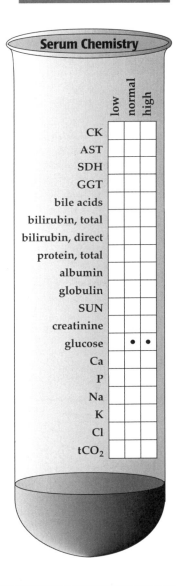

Serum Chemistry

	low	normal	high
CK			
AST			
SDH			
GGT			
bile acids			
bilirubin, total			
bilirubin, direct			
protein, total			
albumin			
globulin			
SUN			
creatinine			
glucose		●	●
Ca			
P			
Na			
K			
Cl			
tCO₂			

Hemogram

	low	normal	high
total RBC			
PCV			
total WBC			
neutrophils	●	●	
bands			
lymphocytes	●	●	
monocytes			
eosinophils			
basophils			
platelets			
fibrinogen			

Urinalysis

	normal	abnormal
color		
blood		
protein		
albumin		
glucose		
pH		
specific gravity		
WBC		
RBC		
epithelial cells		
bacteria		
casts		
crystals		

Special Tests

- ◆ Fluorescent antibody test of brain tissue may be diagnostic for rabies. CSF analysis and serology are characteristic.
- ◆ An increased CSF albumin quotient with normal IgG index is typical of EHV-1 infection (Dr. Frank Andrews, Department of Rural Practice, University of Tennessee, P.O. Box 1071, Knoxville TN, 37901-1071).

● Changes caused by the disease itself

●† Changes secondary to dysfunction caused by the disease

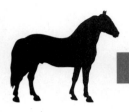

LEUKOENCEPHALOMALACIA

Consumption of feed contaminated with *Fusarium* spp. is the usual cause of leukoencephalomalacia. Clinical signs are usually seen 2 to 3 weeks after ingestion of moldy corn, but it can take up to 24 weeks before any problems are observed. Horses are usually afebrile with signs of cerebral lesions including depression, head-pressing, circling, blindness, and, less frequently, excitement. The disease may progress to recumbency, coma, and death.

INTERPRETATION OF LABORATORY DATA

CSF analysis can show a neutrophilic pleocytosis, but may be normal. Feed samples of stomach contents can be analyzed by thin-layer chromatography or HPLC for the presence of Fumonisin B1 toxin.

The toxin may occasionally cause centrolobular hepatic necrosis, resulting in increases in serum SDH and AST activities. Hemorrhagic enteritis may lead to leukopenia and a left shift. Cystitis with increased urine protein and leukocytes has been noted.

SIGNIFICANT DISEASES TO RULE OUT

◆ Viral myeloencephalitis and encephalomyelitis are diagnosed by interpreting positive titers.
◆ Rabies is diagnosed on postmortem examination of tissues.
◆ Protozoal myeloencephalitis is diagnosed by Western blot analysis of CSF (University of Kentucky).
◆ Verminous or bacterial meningoencephalomyelitis is suspected when viral and protozoal titers are negative.
◆ Brain trauma may present with evidence of hemorrhage in CSF. Viral and protozoal titers are negative. Clinical signs are generally not progressive.

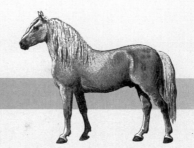

Signs

- Depression
- Circling
- Blindness
- ± Hyper-excitability

Serum Chemistry

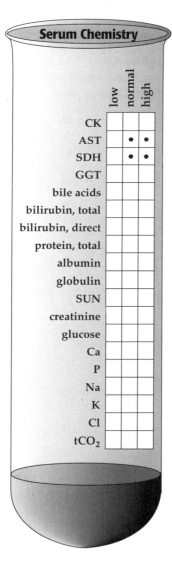

	low	normal	high
CK			
AST		•	•
SDH		•	•
GGT			
bile acids			
bilirubin, total			
bilirubin, direct			
protein, total			
albumin			
globulin			
SUN			
creatinine			
glucose			
Ca			
P			
Na			
K			
Cl			
tCO$_2$			

Hemogram

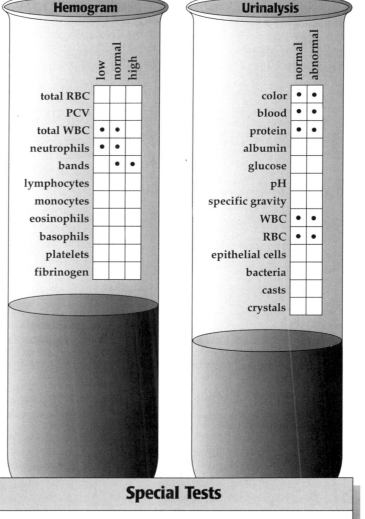

	low	normal	high
total RBC			
PCV			
total WBC	•	•	
neutrophils	•	•	
bands		•	•
lymphocytes			
monocytes			
eosinophils			
basophils			
platelets			
fibrinogen			

Urinalysis

	normal	abnormal
color	•	•
blood	•	•
protein	•	•
albumin		
glucose		
pH		
specific gravity		
WBC	•	•
RBC	•	•
epithelial cells		
bacteria		
casts		
crystals		

Special Tests

- CSF analysis may reveal neutrophilic pleocytosis.
- Necropsy findings are characteristic.
- Feed samples or stomach contents may be positive for the presence of Fumonisin B1 toxin.

- • Changes caused by the disease itself
- •† Changes secondary to dysfunction caused by the disease

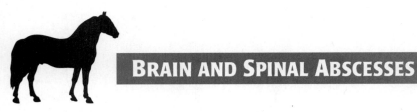

BRAIN AND SPINAL ABSCESSES

Presentation of horses with CNS abscesses varies from few signs or fever to signs of neurologic disease that depend on the location of the lesion. Epizootics of *Streptococcus equi* have been associated with CNS abscesses.

INTERPRETATION OF LABORATORY DATA

Plasma fibrinogen and globulin concentrations and peripheral blood leukocyte counts are increased. Nonregenerative anemia of chronic disease may occur. CSF is usually xanthochromic, with increased protein concentration and possible increased cell counts. A history of *Streptococcus equi* (strangles) aids the diagnosis.

SIGNIFICANT DISEASES TO RULE OUT

Other causes of asymmetric CNS disease:

- ◆ Protozoal myeloencephalitis is diagnosed by Western blot analysis of CSF (University of Kentucky).
- ◆ Verminous or bacterial meningoencephalomyelitis is suspected when viral and protozoal titers are negative.
- ◆ Brain trauma may present with evidence of hemorrhage in CSF. Viral and protozoal titers are negative. Clinical signs are generally not progressive.
- ◆ Cholesterol granuloma is not associated with laboratory data indicative of infection.

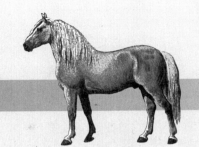

Signs

- Fever
- Ataxia
- Depression
- Circling
- Head-pressing

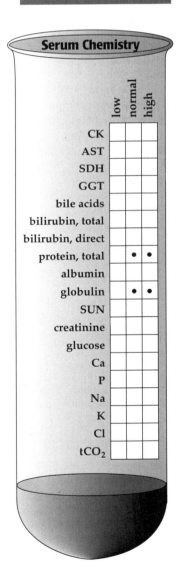

Serum Chemistry

	low	normal	high
CK			
AST			
SDH			
GGT			
bile acids			
bilirubin, total			
bilirubin, direct			
protein, total		•	•
albumin			
globulin		•	•
SUN			
creatinine			
glucose			
Ca			
P			
Na			
K			
Cl			
tCO$_2$			

Hemogram

	low	normal	high
total RBC	•	•	
PCV	•	•	
total WBC			•
neutrophils			•
bands			
lymphocytes			
monocytes			
eosinophils			
basophils			
platelets			
fibrinogen			•

Urinalysis

	normal	abnormal
color		
blood		
protein		
albumin		
glucose		
pH		
specific gravity		
WBC		
RBC		
epithelial cells		
bacteria		
casts		
crystals		

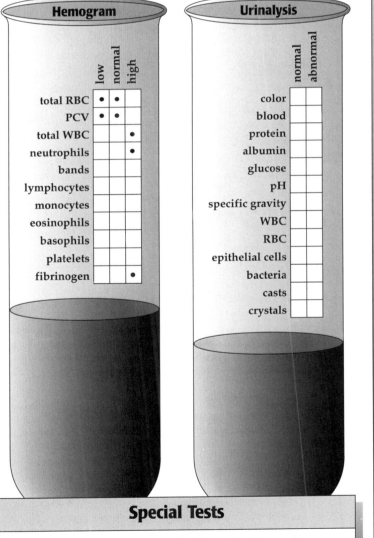

Special Tests

- CSF analysis reveals xanthochromia, elevated protein and cell count.
- Nuclear scintigraphy may reveal a mass.

- Changes caused by the disease itself
- † Changes secondary to dysfunction caused by the disease

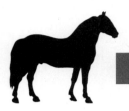

EQUINE PROTOZOAL MYELOENCEPHALITIS

Affected horses often present acutely with no premonitory indication of disease. Early in the course of illness, horses may only appear lame, with later progression to ataxia, spasticity, sweating, reflex loss, cranial nerve dysfunction, recumbency, and muscle atrophy. Signs can be symmetric or asymmetric. The causative agent has been identified as *Sarcocystis falcatula*.

INTERPRETATION OF LABORATORY DATA

CSF analysis is often normal; however, some lesions are large enough to cause xanthochromia, with increases in erythrocytes, protein, and leukocytes (neutrophils). Diagnosis can be made by Western blot and PCR analysis of CSF. Histopathology of the spinal cord reveals the presence of the agent and a necrotizing myelitis with hemorrhage, which is usually bilateral.

SIGNIFICANT DISEASES TO RULE OUT

◆ Verminous or bacterial meningoencephalomyelitis is suspected when viral and protozoal titers in CSF are negative.
◆ Brain trauma may present with evidence of hemorrhage in CSF. Viral and protozoal titers in CSF are negative. Clinical signs are generally not progressive.
◆ Cholesterol granuloma is not associated with laboratory data indicative of infection.
◆ Brain abscess diagnosis is aided by a history of *Streptococcus equi* (strangles).

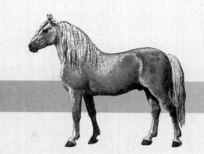

Signs

- ◆ Ataxia
- ◆ Apparent lameness
- ◆ Sweating
- ◆ Reflex loss
- ◆ Spasticity
- ◆ Muscle atrophy

Serum Chemistry

	low	normal	high
CK			
AST			
SDH			
GGT			
bile acids			
bilirubin, total			
bilirubin, direct			
protein, total			
albumin			
globulin			
SUN			
creatinine			
glucose			
Ca			
P			
Na			
K			
Cl			
tCO$_2$			

Hemogram

	low	normal	high
total RBC			
PCV			
total WBC			
neutrophils			
bands			
lymphocytes			
monocytes			
eosinophils			
basophils			
platelets			
fibrinogen			

Urinalysis

	normal	abnormal
color		
blood		
protein		
albumin		
glucose		
pH		
specific gravity		
WBC		
RBC		
epithelial cells		
bacteria		
casts		
crystals		

Special Tests

- ◆ Western blot analysis of CSF (Equine Biodiagnostics, Q165 ASTeCC Building, University of Kentucky, Lexington, KY 40506-0286) will reveal antibody to *Sarcocystis falcatula*. PCR may reveal protozoal DNA.
- ◆ CSF protein electrophoresis may reveal normal albumin quotient and elevated IgG index indicative of intrathecal production of immunoglobulin. (Dr. Frank Andrews, Department of Rural Practice, University of Tennessee, P.O. Box 1071, Knoxville TN, 37901-1071)

• Changes caused by the disease itself
•† Changes secondary to dysfunction caused by the disease

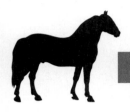

MENINGITIS

Bacterial meningitis in foals occurs as a complication of septicemia and is an uncommon cause of cerebral disease in adults. Clinical signs include fever and hyperesthesia followed by depression, aimless walking, behavioral changes, abnormal vocalization, and seizures.

INTERPRETATION OF LABORATORY DATA

Dehydrated foals may develop metabolic derangements of azotemia and hypoglycemia. The CBC reflects evidence of sepsis with neutropenia and a left shift in acute stages. Neutrophilia and hyperfibrinogenemia occur later in the disease process. The presence of bacteria and increased numbers of leukocytes (neutrophils) and protein concentration in CSF is diagnostic; however, the absence of bacteria does not rule out sepsis. CSF and blood should be cultured. In adults, CSF changes may be the only abnormal finding.

SIGNIFICANT DISEASES TO RULE OUT

- ◆ Neonatal maladjustment syndrome reveals a normal CSF with a normal leukocyte count.
- ◆ Other cerebral diseases in adults do not reveal the characteristic findings of meningitis.

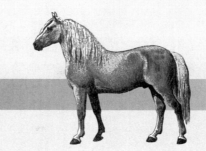

Signs

- ◆ Fever
- ◆ Depression
- ◆ Hyperesthesia
- ◆ Behavioral change
- ◆ Abnormal vocalization

Serum Chemistry

	low	normal	high
CK			
AST			
SDH			
GGT			
bile acids			
bilirubin, total			
bilirubin, direct			
protein, total			
albumin			
globulin			
SUN		•	•
creatinine		•	•
glucose	•	•	
Ca			
P			
Na			
K			
Cl			
tCO$_2$			

Hemogram

	low	normal	high
total RBC			
PCV			
total WBC	•	•	•
neutrophils	•	•	•
bands		•	•
lymphocytes			
monocytes			
eosinophils			
basophils			
platelets			
fibrinogen		•	•

Urinalysis

	normal	abnormal
color		
blood		
protein		
albumin		
glucose		
pH		
specific gravity		
WBC		
RBC		
epithelial cells		
bacteria		
casts		
crystals		

Special Tests

- ◆ CSF analysis will reveal increased cells (neutrophils), protein, and, in severe cases, bacteria.

- • Changes caused by the disease itself
- •† Changes secondary to dysfunction caused by the disease

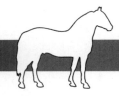

P, Q

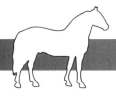

G

O